AF118914

THE ART OF

BELLY DANCE

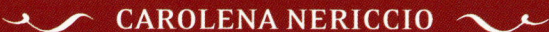

A Fun and Fabulous Way to Get Fit

∼ CAROLENA NERICCIO ∼

becker&mayer!BOOKS

Bellevue, Washington

Copyright © 2004 by Carolena Nericcio

All rights reserved. No part of this book may be reproduced in any form without written permission from the publisher.

ISBN: 1-932855-04-1

PRINTED IN CHINA

AUDIO/DVD COORDINATION: Kate Hall
DESIGN: Joanna Price
EDITORIAL: Adrienne Wiley
PRODUCTION COORDINATION: Sheila Hackler
PROJECT MANAGEMENT: Sheila Kamuda

10 9 8 7 6 5 4 3 2 1

becker&mayer! Books
11010 Northup Way
Bellevue, Washington 98004

www.beckermayer.com

CONTENTS

· · · · · · · · · · · · · · · ·

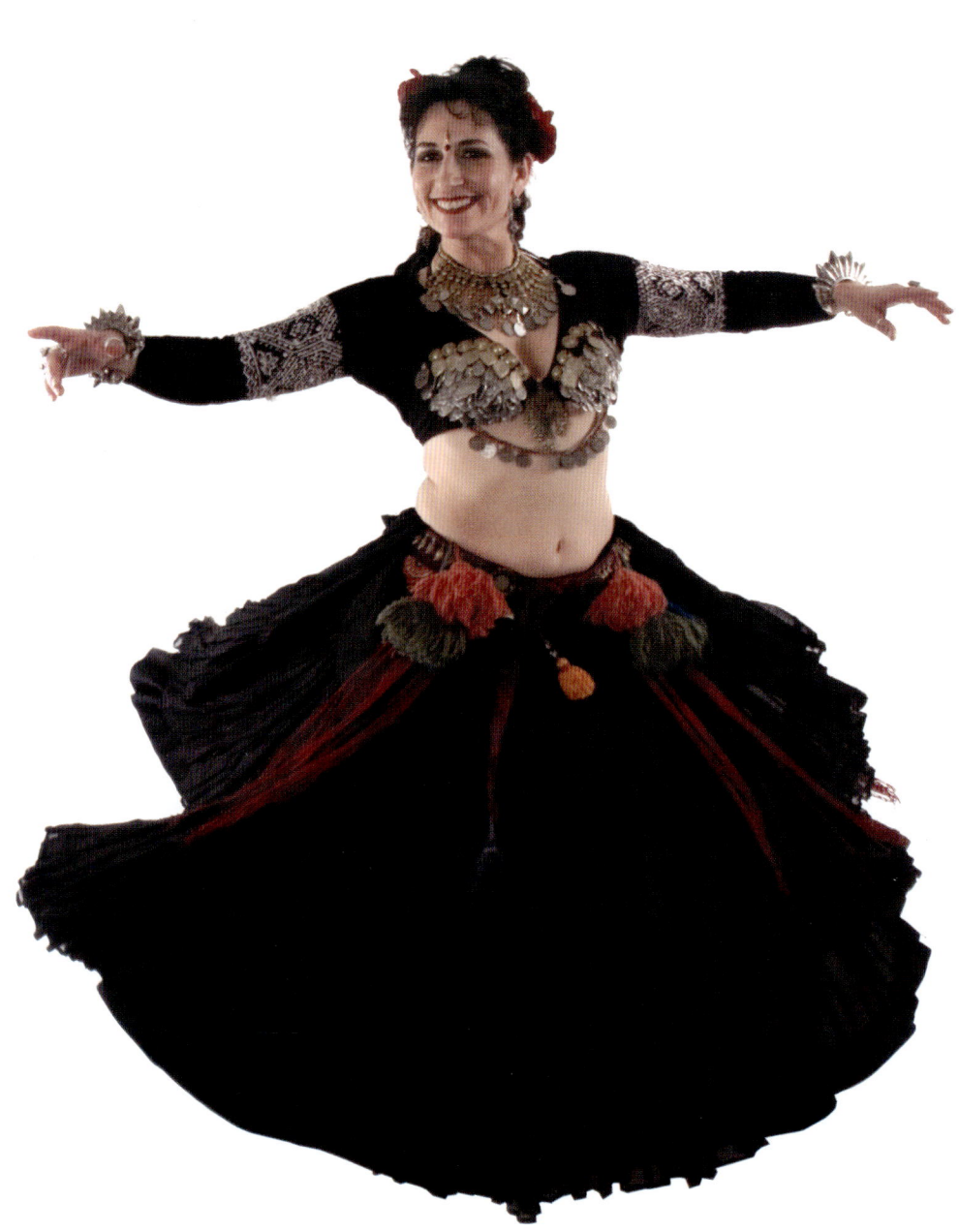

INTRODUCTION
The Shimmy Is the Bounce in a Healthy Woman's Step

Sometimes when I'm presenting the shimmy to a new group of dancers, I see them get that glazed look that says, "I don't get it." This is my favorite challenge: how to present a concept so that everyone can understand. I can tell you the mechanics of how the shimmy works, I can tell you how it fits into the music, I can tell you where it goes in the choreography, but sometimes a dancer needs a visualization to make the connection.

So I say, "Imagine this: there was a time in history, a long time ago, when the bounce and sway of a woman's hips was considered so beautiful they set it to music and made a dance out of it."

I tell my students to put their hands on their hips and simply walk around the room. You can feel the fat and muscle reach, contract, and reverberate with each step, the same way every time. A woman's hips are *supposed* to bounce. Set it to rhythmic music, and you've got the beginning of a dance.

But what happened to that time and place? How did we go from honoring the natural shape and substance of a woman's body to seeing it as something imperfect? Nature created us perfectly—an incredible system of nerves, muscle, bone, and blood, all interwoven in such a way that an impulse from the brain can make a hip bounce or an eyelash flutter. The modern culture in which we live has no interest in the original perfection of the body. We seem to have lost our respect for nature and its infinite wisdom of balance.

I'm not saying that we should just sit down and eat bonbons in front of the television, expecting the world to drop by and tell us we're beautiful just the way we are. What I'm saying is we could do more for ourselves by accepting what we've been given. Recognize the parts that work and make them your assets, then acknowledge the parts that you want to change and work to make them stronger.

I chose belly dance when I was fourteen because I was too shy to dance with boys. I wanted to be able to enjoy moving to music whenever I wanted to, without having to wait for someone to ask me to join him. At fourteen, I wasn't interested in fitness. Another byproduct of being shy, I failed at team sports and felt uncomfortable about my big hips. I had no idea you could change things like body image, confidence, a charismatic smile. I saw belly dance as a solo activity. Ironically, I chose a dance of presentation. Shyness became stage presence, big hips became bouncing hips, the desire to dance by myself transformed into the pleasure of sharing the dance with others. I became so transfixed by the balance and power of the body that I became a personal trainer as well as a dance teacher and professional performer.

Whatever your reason for learning the art of belly dance, remember that belly dance is about feminine beauty. The shape and meaning of the dance display the strength and beauty of the female body. Dancing alone in front of the mirror, you are still using the gestures of presentation. Dancing with a partner, you reflect her beauty. Dancing for an audience, you are the mirror of their feeling for the music.

Whether you choose belly dance as a physical activity, a mental challenge, or an emotional release, mastering the steps can provide a sense of well being and satisfaction. One doesn't need prior dance experience or special conditioning before learning to dance. Belly dance is gentle by nature, and you can decide how vigorously you want to approach it. However, it is always wise to consult your physician if you have any questions.

In this book you will find warm-up exercises, the basic steps and gestures of belly dance, a simple section on music and costume ideas, and loads of encouragement.

Thank you for joining me. I hope you enjoy the dance as much as I do.

THE HISTORY OF BELLY DANCE

The movement art known in the West as belly dance has existed for thousands of years, although it continues to evolve even today.

This thousand-year history can be viewed in two different ways. The first interprets belly dance as a dance done only in the company of other women. Traditional Islam, the prevailing religion in belly dance's lands of origin, restricts a woman's contact with people outside her immediate household and family. Therefore, before the advent of radio and television as means of entertainment, women would gather together in their houses and courtyards to help each other with daily chores or to talk and relax when the work was done. Singing, dancing, and storytelling were the entertainments of choice. Out of these gatherings came this playful and flirtatious dance. It consists largely of bouncing and shimmying hips, delicate hand and arm gestures, and fluid and sinewy undulations of the body, all of which were passed on as young girls watched older women dance. Where did the original movements come from? That's an answer we'd all like to have! Perhaps it was a form of storytelling, perhaps pillow talk for a new bride. The result is a very feminine dance that cele-brates life and delights in the shape and display of the female body.

The second interpretation of the dance is as a part of the role of the professional entertainer. Professional entertainers were not bound by the rules of Islam regarding a woman's activities, and so could display these sensual dances outside the home and to any audience. Originally, these women may have been Gypsies or other itinerant travelers, or simply women who, because of financial woes, were forced to work outside the home, thus forfeiting their status as "respectable women."

Modern belly dance, however practiced or danced, draws from both of these histories. It has blossomed out of North Africa and is enjoyed all over the world.

American Tribal Style Belly Dance

There are several elements that distinguish American Tribal Style belly dance, the style I typically teach, from other styles of belly dance. From its name we learn two of the most important. *American* identifies this style as a modern fusion of many dancing traditions. *Tribal Style* refers to its appearance when performed, with several women dressed in layers of costume and jewelry dancing together.

That the dance is designed for group performance is significant. The steps and gestures are simple and uniform so that two, three, or four dancers at a time can easily assimilate cues and gestures. The uniformity isn't intended to eliminate a dancer's individuality, but rather allows her uniqueness to enhance the overall impact of the performance. Different body heights, weights, and shapes appear in step together on the stage, providing a visual array of beauty.

The steps and movements of Tribal Style have evolved from both Egyptian Cabaret and the folkloric dances of North Africa, as well as inheriting some stylistic influences from the Spanish Flamenco and the dances of India. More generally, Tribal steps are derived from everyday gestures, so the audience often unconsciously "connects" to the dance through our collective muscle memory. The dance form is constantly evolving, and to this day we keep our eyes and ears open and are always adding to our repertoire. Tribal is also a largely improvisational style of belly dance, using simple steps and gestures in a repetitive fashion, building on the music and the interaction between the dancers.

The musical choices of Tribal Style are also unique. We favor Egyptian Folkloric music over Classical Arabic because of the repetitive nature of its phrasing. Classical Arabic music is designed for one dancer interacting with the musicians and the audience. Folkloric is traditionally performed for a group dancing together, often for long periods of time. We find the Folkloric music gives us time to set up a movement, repeat it several times, and make a change, all within one phrase. We do use other types of music as well, including other Middle Eastern and African Folkloric songs, as well as some contemporary fusions such as Rai and World Beat. In choosing the music, we are always looking for the distinctive *taxeem*–the slow, improvisational sections of the song–and the driving, up-tempo beat, which encourages the more lively steps.

The costume also distinguishes Tribal. A typical Tribal costume consists of pantaloons, a full skirt, a hip shawl, and a *choli* (open-backed shirt). For performance, we often add a coin bra, a tassel belt or coin sash, and a headdress or hair swept up and adorned with flowers. Opulent displays of jewelry, such as coin necklaces, bracelets and cuffs, rings, and ornaments pinned anywhere that might catch the eye or enhance movement are also encouraged. There is no "right" or "wrong" way to put together a costume, as long as it empowers the wearer by flattering the line of the body and augments the display of steps and gestures.

Despite the differences between styles, it is most important to remember that belly dance is belly dance the world over. Its main attraction is delight. The dancer feels good doing it, and the audience takes pleasure in watching it.

GETTING STARTED

Fitness

Physical activity is too often looked upon as a chore. But dancing is physical activity we enjoy. Why? Is it the music, the companionship, the satisfaction of learning a new step or sequence? All of these things are nice, but more likely it's that dancing— moving—makes us feel good. When we exercise, more oxygen is called for as the brain and muscles burn up the resting reserve. Also, endorphins are released as the body senses the extra work at hand, a useful trait inherited from our hunter-gatherer ancestors. The result is a boost in mood and energy.

Is belly dance an aerobic activity? Yes and no. When we dance for the art of it, we are creating a varied landscape by changing the steps appropriately with the music. This variation also serves to switch muscle groups, which keeps the dance from becoming a typical workout.

However, any new activity is a challenge until the body gets used to the routine. This doesn't mean that an activity loses its usefulness; it means that your body has found a way to approach it more efficiently. Your body doesn't know that you are trying to burn fat or build muscle; it is just protecting its hard-won calories and water by minimizing the effort needed for the task at hand—the hunter-gatherer thing again.

When you first begin dancing, your body may treat the up-tempo steps as aerobic and the slow movements as isometric or toning. As you progress, you will develop the ability to make the steps and movements aerobic *and* toning, or apparently effortless. Repeating the same step or movement over and over will cause it to become an exercise, while varying the movement or changing from fast to slow choreography will make the dance appear effortless.

Belly dance can be a medium-level aerobic exercise if you use the up-tempo steps in a repetitive fashion. If you want to try this, pick an upbeat piece of music that will run for at least twenty minutes (such as tracks 5–10 on the enclosed CD). With respect to the broad changes in the music, stay with one movement (or, better yet, the whole family of movements) for as long as you can. Warm up with *taxeem* and slow movements. Progress to a fast pace, then cool down with more *taxeem* and some easy stretches. Use as much overhead arm placement as possible, as this helps to raise the heart rate. Allow the steps and movements to sink in, and push them harder than you would if you were performing. I think you'll be pleased with the results.

The Belly

There are common misconceptions that belly dance will make the belly either larger or smaller. Indeed, your belly may take on a new shape as you begin to dance. The posture and movements will lengthen and strengthen the back and condition the abdomen, including the obliques (see sidebar). The result will be a more shapely midsection with no abnormal change in your belly's shape.

OBLIQUES

The obliques are the muscles of the abdomen. They run in a criss-cross fashion along the sides of the torso. There are two sets of obliques: the internal and the external. The internal originate at the back hip and insert at the lower front ribcage. The external originate at the lower front ribcage and insert at the front hip. The obliques are responsible for side bending and turning or twisting at the waist. As we progress, you'll begin to see how important the obliques are to our dance. Also, when the obliques are toned, they effectively serve to "winch" the waist.

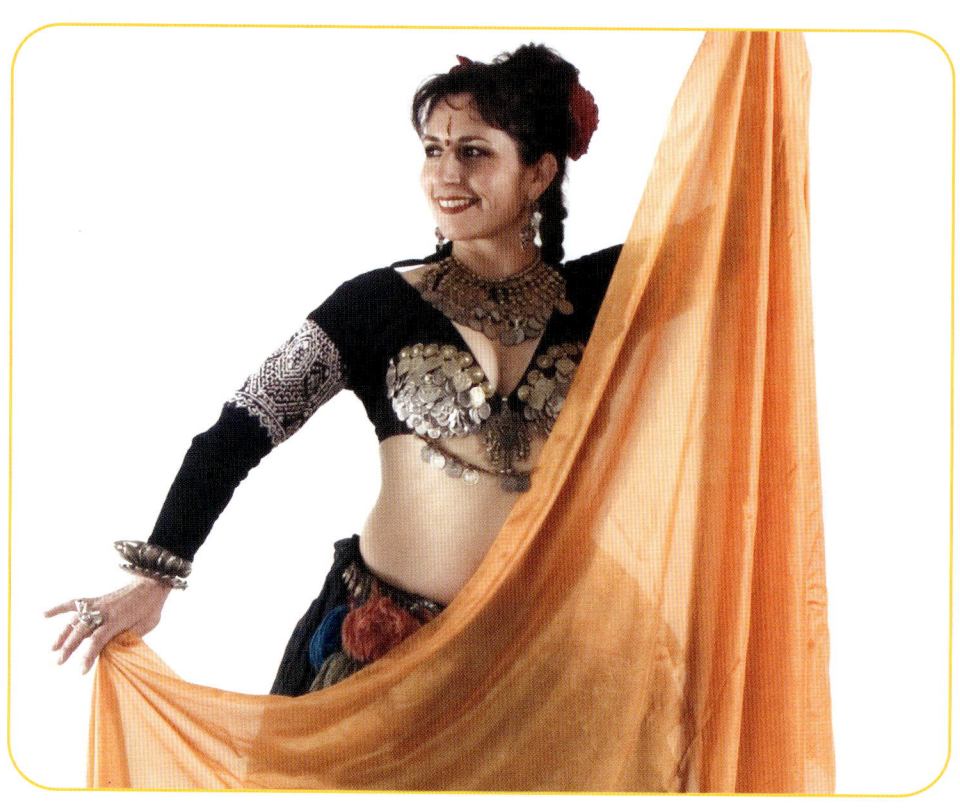

A Note About Progress

Everyone learns at a different pace. If you practice every week, you will have a good understanding of what's going on within a few months. Obviously, if you devote more than one day a week, you'll move along faster than if you start and stop.

Every now and then you'll reach a plateau. At these points it may feel as if you've been working at the same thing forever and are not making progress. This is natural. You may be overdoing it, or you may be trying to push a movement in the wrong direction. In either case, take a break. Let your brain and body have a rest, and you'll be able to go back to the dance with a refreshed attitude and enthusiasm.

THE COSTUME

As described earlier, the typical Tribal costume is a visually elaborate collection of jewelry, long scarves, and flowing skirts. However, it's not necessary to purchase any kind of fantastic costume for practice. You'll want to wear something that allows a full range of motion. Tights and a *choli* (open-backed shirt) or leotard are fine. Add a hip shawl for a feeling of definition and flair at the hip, and you're ready to go.

If you want to put together a more elaborate costume, you can follow some of our makeup and costuming tips. Our skirts measure a full ten yards at the hem, with adjustable elastic at the hip. This allows for a full range of motion and helps define the sweeping motion of the movements. You can purchase a skirt or make your own, with a wide enough hem to give you the freedom to move without restriction. Our skirts fall just above the floor. We like the aesthetic line it gives the body, but if you feel you might trip over something that long, by all means, choose your own length!

Below the skirt we wear pantaloons to cover the legs. Our pantaloons are a full four yards of fabric gathered at the ankle and feature an elastic hip and dropped crotch. We then tie a shawl or scarf around the hips. This hip scarf is the most classic of all belly dance attire. It serves to accentuate the hips to both the observer and the wearer. Our shawls have fringe for added movement.

On top, we wear a *choli,* a modified version of the midriff blouses worn under Indian saris. They are snug-fitting but not restrictive, and can be worn without a bra. Our *cholis* have open backs and gussets at the underarm to accommodate overhead movement. Ties at the neck and mid-back make fitting easy.

The headdress is not, as some onlookers presume, a pre-made hat. The headdress is a series of layered scarves, created each time it is worn and decorated with jewelry and flowers. The base is a large scarf or piece of fabric, roughly 45 x 90 . This base is wrapped around the head and built up to form a "platform" for the smaller accent scarves. We then add flowers and jewelry to flatter and frame the face. Everything is either tied securely or pinned with safety and hat pins.

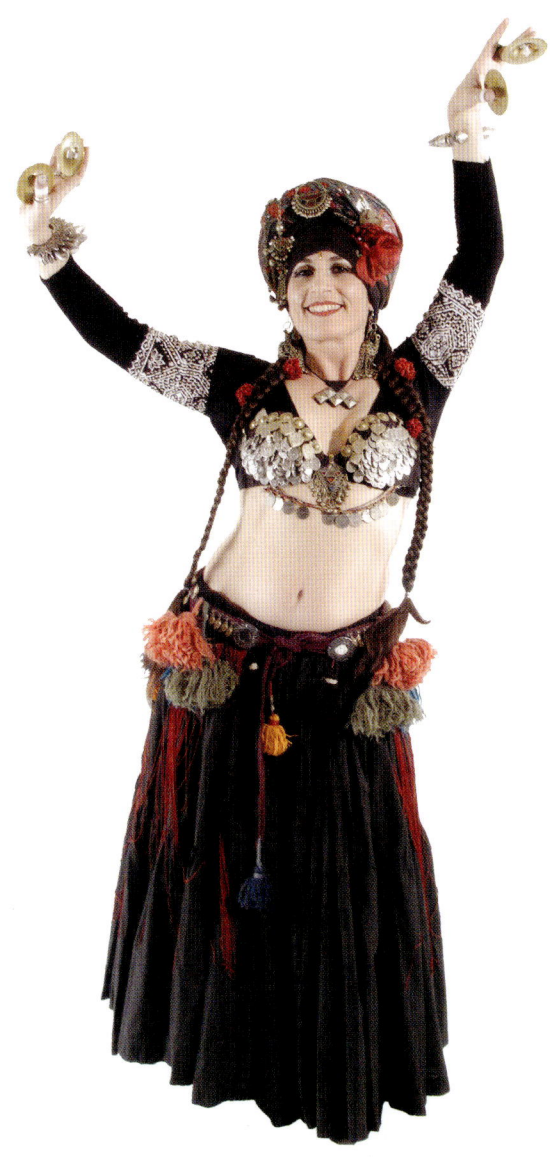

THE MUSIC

One of the most important aspects of any style of belly dance is the dancer's ability to interpret the music. It is here that things begin to connect. The musician plays, and the dancer listens to the music and displays what she feels; the audience experiences both the sound and the movement. A perfect example of the collective unconscious—everyone is participating in the event. It's really a phenomenon: through music played by one person and movement danced by another, the complete sensation can be felt by a third person. The oldest form of virtual reality! In an atmosphere sympathetic to the history of the dance, the emotional reaction this elicits is almost always accompanied by a *zaghareet,* a shrill trilling, from both the performers and the audience.

Arabic music is a science in and of itself, and we can't do justice to it in this humble book. What follows is a brief overview of some of the instruments and rhythms used in the music that accompanies Tribal Style. Note that spellings vary, as the common names are usually phonetic translations of the Arabic; in fact, some will have several wholly different names as there are regional differences in what they are called.

The Instruments

PERCUSSION:

· Doumbec, Darbukka, Arabic Tabla: A goblet-shaped drum made of clay or metal. Traditionally, the head of this drum was an animal or fish skin stretched across the upper end. The Doumbec is played with the hands and fingertips. The "doum" sound comes from beating the hand on the center of the drum. The "bec" (or "tek," as it is more often known) is played by hitting the edge of the drum.

- Def, Duff, Tar: A shallow-frame drum, similar in look to a tambourine without cymbals. The Def is played with the hand and fingertips. A variety of sounds can be achieved—some dry and airy, some distinct.
- Bendir: A frame drum similar to the Def, but with strings suspended across the inside to create a reverberation. The sound is similar to the Def, but the strings give it an added "buzz."
- Riqq: An Arabic tambourine with a fish skin or Mylar head. The frame is often inlaid with mother of pearl in a very ornate geometric pattern. Held in an upright position, primary sounds are made by tapping the fingertips on both the head and the cymbals, and through a series of shakes and combinations. Small as it is, the Riqq is the lead percussion instrument.
- Muzhar: Looking like a large tambourine, the Muzhar adds dimension and drama to the music. It sounds a bit like thunder and rain. As with the Riqq, it is primarily played upright with the hand and fingertips.
- Tabla Beledi, Tapan, Davul: The base drum. It looks a lot like a typical base drum, with two heads and a laced body, but the Tabla Beledi is hung around the shoulder with a strap so the heads fall to the right and left rather than up and down. The musician uses a club and switch and sometimes hands to make a variety of sounds. The Tabla Beledi adds texture and depth to the simplest arrangements.
- Zils, Sagat, Finger Cymbals: Four small circles of metal. A hole or slot in the top of the Zils allows them to be affixed to the thumb and middle fingers of each hand with a small piece of elastic. The Zils are played by tapping the thumb and middle finger together. (See pages 72-76 for more information.)

MELODY:

- Mizmar, Zourna, Ghaita: A double-reed instrument similar to an oboe. The Mizmar is *loud* and rarely needs amplification. Used almost exclusively for Folkloric music, the Mizmar can be both melodic and rhythmic. A Mizmar player will often keep time with the percussionist. At times, you might even find yourself following the Mizmar for tempo rather than the drum.

- Nai, Ney, Nay: A flute made from reeds that grow along the Nile, the Nai is one of the simplest and most fragile instruments. The finger holes are drilled first, and then the whole thing is hollowed out. It has no other components except the finger holes and the breath that blows into it. It sounds like a sigh.
- Accordion: Although not originally from Egypt, the Accordion has become a standard instrument, playing either harmony or melody.
- Oud, Ud: A stringed instrument played with a plectrum (similar to a pick). The Oud has a deep, round body with a hole in the center and a short neck to which eleven strings are attached. The Oud is very soft and is easily drowned out by other instruments.
- Rebaba: A stick fiddle with two strings, played vertically with a bow made of Egyptian horsehair. A simple Rebaba might be made by stretching a fish skin over half of a coconut shell or tuna can! The sound is often mistaken for a wind instrument. It holds a strong, steady note.
- Arghool, Arghul: The Arghool is a single-reed instrument, made of two pipes bound together and played at the same time. The shorter of the two plays the melody; the longer holds down a "drone" sound. The Arghool brings intensity and anticipation to the music.

The Rhythms

There are dozens of rhythms in the world of Arabic music, but the standard structure of Tribal Style music is simple. By sticking to a basic format, we can easily connect the steps to the rhythms. Common rhythms include:

- Fallahi, Ayoob, Malfuf, Karachi: variations of two counts.
- Baladi (Maqsoum, Masmoudi Saghira, Saaidi): variations of four counts.
- Chiftitelli, Masmoudi: variations of eight counts.

More often than not, a rhythm is grouped in phrases of four measures. So, a dancer can anticipate that a musician will most likely play three measures identically, vary the fourth, and then switch to another tempo, beat, or melodic phrase.

Dancing to the Music

Whether fast or slow, the most prized Tribal Style music has long sections of repetitive phrases, with a melody that can be a decorative drum pattern, vocals, or a melody instrument.

A solo dancer may choose to move quickly between the subtle changes in the music, but as an improvisational duet or trio, the application changes. For the magic of improvisation the dancers need time to play out the cues and transitions. Even with choreography, the group needs time to create the feeling of a wave lapping gently or crashing against the shore.

How we choose to use the music is dictated by the source, history, feeling, and shape of the song. And take it from me: if a musician feels you aren't responding to what he is playing, he can make your dance fall flat. So in order to ensure a happy musician, learn about the music you are dancing to!

When you stand on stage the audience should get the feeling that the music is cascading down, over, and around you. There is no movement until you reach out and grab a note, hold it until just the right moment, and then release it.

There is a CD included in this package that features thirteen tracks selected to illustrate this concept. You'll find four slow pieces, three medium-fast pieces, and two fast pieces. We've also included "Baladi Unplugged," a teaching track created for me by Helm, which accelerates in tempo. We find it's great when you are ready to challenge yourself. Lastly, we have a full dance suite that you can use with your own inspiration or our choreography notes on pages 85-94.

WARM-UP STRETCHES

Try to stretch a little bit everyday. You can use the stretches described here, or you can improvise with an intuitive stretching sequence. Just "follow the stretch" around your body until you feel like you've chased the tension away. Your dance will benefit from fluid, flexible muscles.

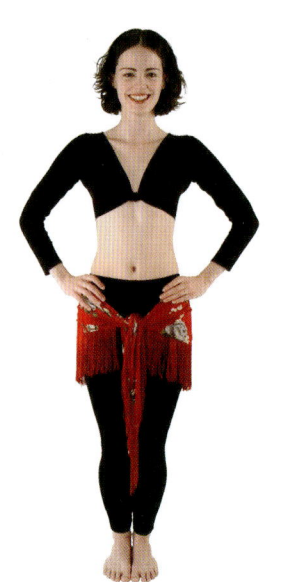

STEP 1

With your feet flat on the floor, bring your heels as close together as is comfortable. Soften your knees, and rock your weight back into your heels. Roll your shoulders back and down, letting your ribcage lift in front. Lastly, release your lower back by contracting slightly at the lower abdomen. (This stance is covered in detail in the posture section beginning on page 24.)

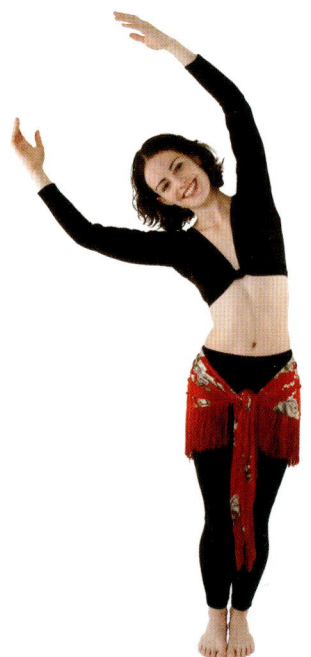

STEP 2

Bring your arms overhead. Stay focused on your center. Lower yourself over to one side. Your spine should be a smooth, even arc, and your weight should be distributed equally on your feet. As you return to center, engage your obliques to keep the pressure out of your lower back. Repeat on the other side, and then repeat this several times. Back at center, bring your arms back down.

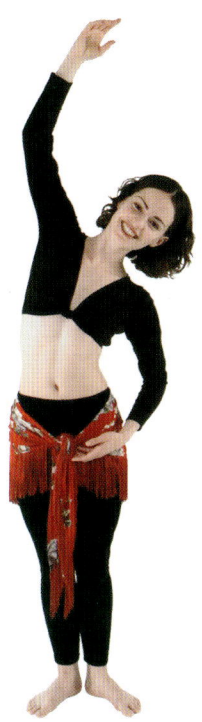

STEP 3

Reach up with one arm and down with the other, as if you are pulling your fingertips apart. Let your arms come back to center as you return to your starting position. Repeat on the other side. Now, take a deep breath as you repeat the sequence and return to the starting position.

STEP 4

Lift your arms overhead again, grasping your hands and pulling against your own strength. Pull your elbows back behind your ears, open your ribcage, and let your hips hang from your spine. Switch your grip, and repeat. Gently release your arms.

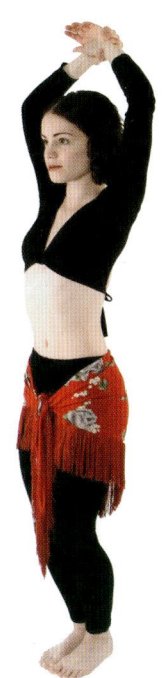

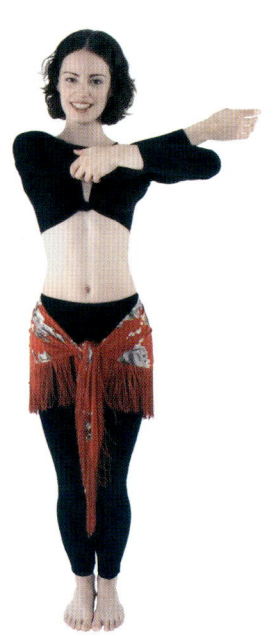

STEP 5

Draw one arm across your chest, and use the other arm to pull back, opening the back and shoulder. Wiggle your fingers to release the tension in your arm. Repeat with the other arm.

STEP 6

Take half a step forward with one foot and a big step back with the other. Keeping your back leg straight and your spine vertical, bend the front leg until you feel a good stretch in the hip flexor of the long back leg. Sink into this stretch, while keeping your spine straight.

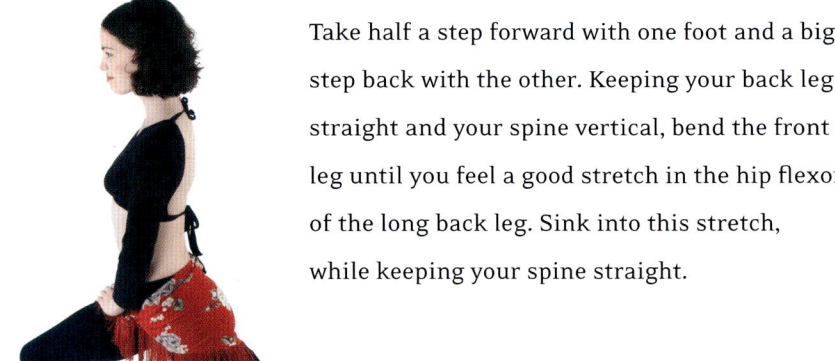

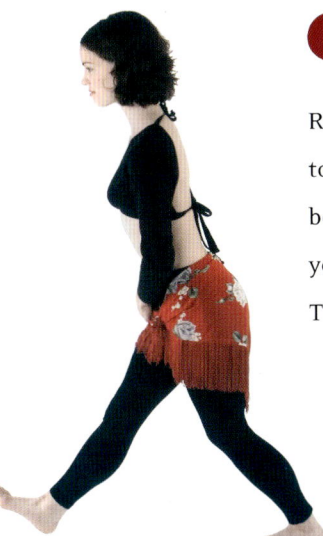

STEP 7

Rock your weight onto the back leg and lift the toes of the front foot. Keep your back flat, and bend at the waist to stretch your hamstrings. Put your toes down, and return to an upright position. Then repeat steps 6 and 7 on the other side.

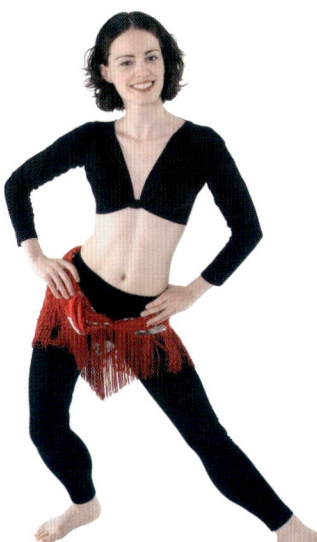

STEP 8

Stand with your feet at shoulder's width, with your hands on your hips for balance. Shift your weight to the right leg, flex your knees, and pull your pelvis down and around until your weight is on your left leg. Continue drawing an "O" with your hips, circling from right to left, then change directions and shift from left to right.

POSTURE

· · · · · · · · · · · · · · · · ·

The spine is designed to support the weight of the body without putting any additional strain on the muscles. However, your daily posture favors your upper body, relying on a slight curve at your tailbone for stability. For this kind of dance, however, we want to shift that stability to the ribcage, leaving the tailbone free to move.

This ribcage lift is sometimes mistaken for an arch in the low back. This is not the case. In lifting the ribcage and releasing the tailbone, we are trying to spare the low back by taking the tension out of it. This dance posture may feel awkward at first, but the more you use it, the better your back will feel and the more freedom of movement you will have.

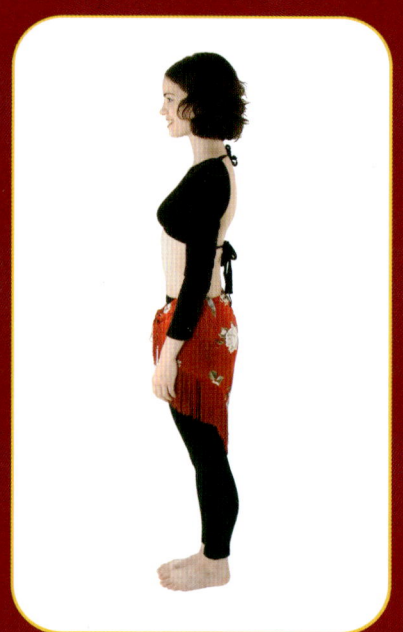

DAILY POSTURE

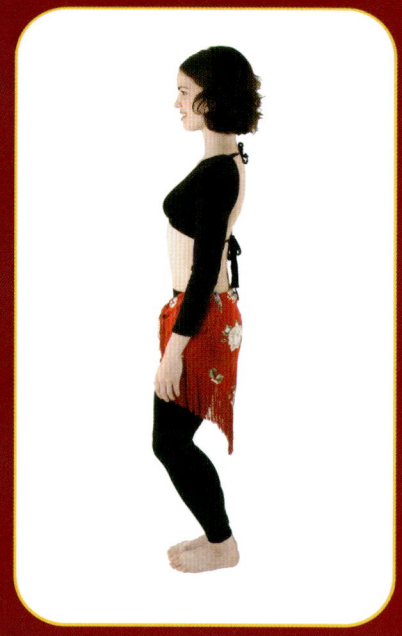

DANCE POSTURE

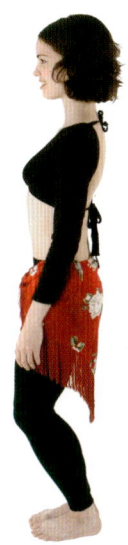

STEP 1

With your feet flat, bring your heels as close together as is comfortable. Soften your knees by flexing gently to create a cushion. Let your tailbone release by slightly contracting the lower abdominal. This should take the pressure out of your lower back. It will feel as if your weight is in your heels.

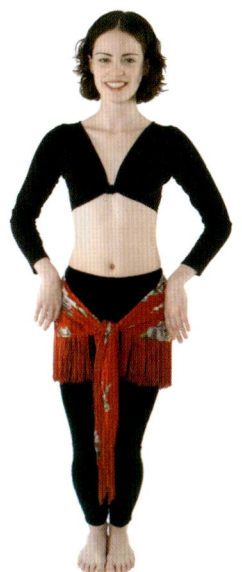

STEP 2

Lift the front of your ribcage by rolling your shoulders back and down and sliding the shoulder blades straight down. Now contract the muscles in the middle of your back. You should feel support from behind and an openness in the front. You are, in effect, standing behind your center.

STEP 3

The shape of the arm is always a soft curve. This is accomplished by holding the shoulder down as you lift the elbow up. When the arm is resting at the hip, the shoulder is down and the elbow is forward. When the arm is lifted to the side, the shoulder is down and the elbow is up. When the arm is overhead, the shoulder is down and the elbow is back.

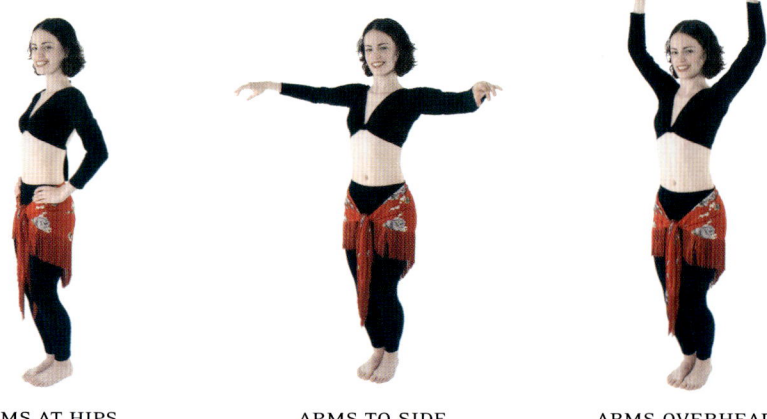

ARMS AT HIPS   ARMS TO SIDE   ARMS OVERHEAD

If correct posture still eludes you, try this exercise. Lie on your back with your knees bent and your feet flat. Reach under your lower back. You will feel a gap between your back and the floor. Some people can slide their hand into the gap; others might have only enough room for a fingertip.

Now, to feel the lower abdominal contraction that creates dance posture, pull your lower back flat to the floor *without* pressing your feet into the floor or contracting your glutei. You might have to relax and try several times, but eventually you will be able to isolate your lower abdominal and pull your lower back flat.

Stand up and repeat this exercise, but this time as if you were pulling the lower back toward the wall. Don't tuck your hips by contracting the glutei or tightening the thighs. The effect you are after is not so much that the back be flat as that the lower back release.

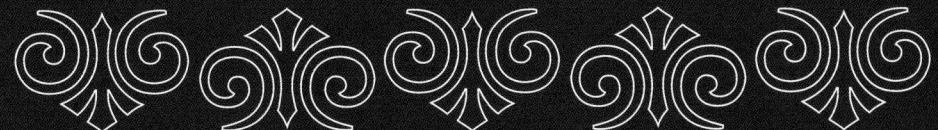

MOVING MEDITATION

Each time I come to dance, I find it appropriate to perform a moving meditation. This meditation is loosely based on the *Puja* performed by Indian dancers before each class or performance they participate in. For me it carries no religious significance but seeks to acknowledge all of the elements that bring me to dance.

STEP 1

Stand with your feet as close together as is comfortable, in dance posture.

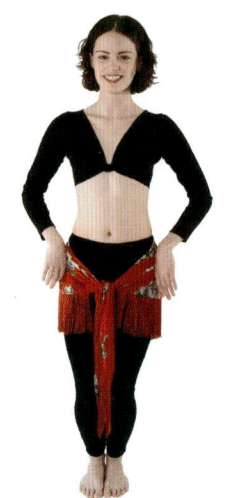

STEP 2

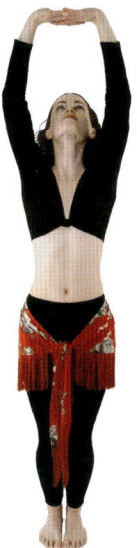

Bring your arms overhead and lace your fingers together, palms facing the ceiling. Stretch the arms and ribcage up and away from the hips. Take a deep breath. Exhale as you release the arms and bring them out to the side, elbows lifted.

STEP 3

Bend the arms so that your hands are placed in front of your chest, palms down, index fingers touching. This position shows that you are preparing to make a gesture from your heart.

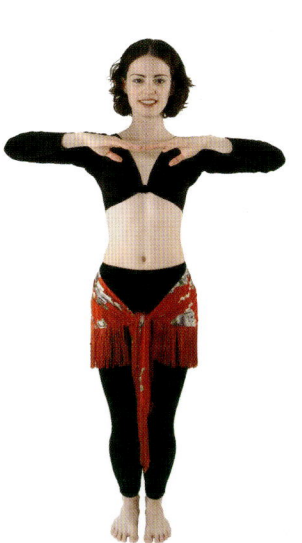

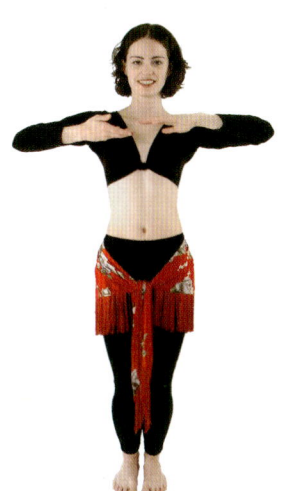

STEP 4

Without dropping the elbow, rotate the wrist and turn the right palm up with your pinky finger closest to your chest, as if you were holding something on the flat of your hand.

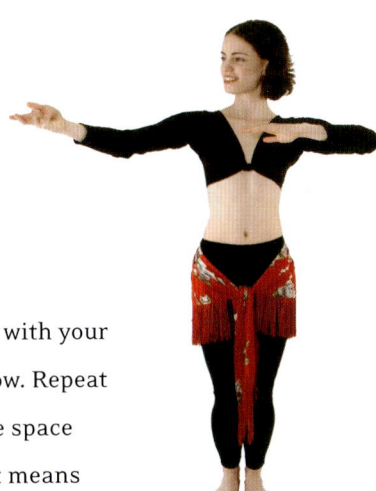

STEP 5

Sweep through the front and right diagonal with your right hand and forearm, pivoting at the elbow. Repeat with the left. This gesture acknowledges the space that you are dancing in, whether to you that means the studio or room, the entire Earth, or all the spaces you have danced in.

STEP 6

Next is the Lotus Blossom, which symbolizes the ongoing nature of life. With your hands in "heart gesture" position as in step 4, let the left palm fall toward your body and the right palm fall out.

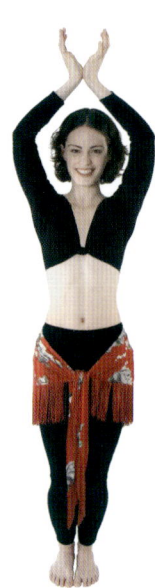

STEP 7

Bring both hands overhead, through your center, as if you were tracing the stem of the lotus with the thumb and index finger of each hand. When you reach the top, form the Lotus Blossom by touching the base of both wrists, palms facing center.

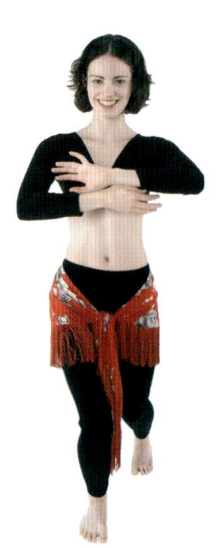

STEP 8

Close the blossom by reversing the ascent of the hand, right palm falling toward your body, left palm falling out. Then, bring both hands through the center as you crouch down on one knee.

STEP 9

Let your hands fall apart naturally as you look at the floor and touch the floor with your fingertips. This gesture acknowledges the surface that you dance on.

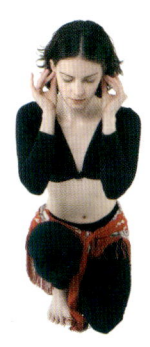

STEP 10

Keep your gaze on the floor. Reach up, and touch the lobe of each ear with your thumb and forefinger. This gesture acknowledges the music that you dance to. Touch the floor again.

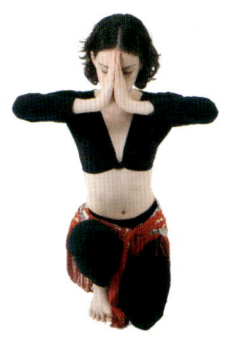

STEP 11

Keeping your gaze on the floor, bring the hands together, palms facing, and touch your forehead with the outside edges of the index fingers. This gesture acknowledges your teachers.

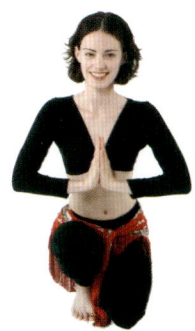

STEP 12

Look up, and bring your facing palms to your heart. This gesture acknowledges your ancestors, dancing or otherwise.

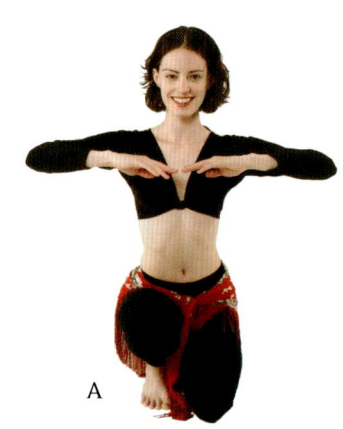

A

Now come back to the original heart position: elbows lifted, palms down, index fingers touching (A). Finally, collect all of the elements as you stand up. Drop the hands (B), and sweep out to the sides and up overhead (C). End by bringing both palms facing at "heart position," elbows lifted (D).

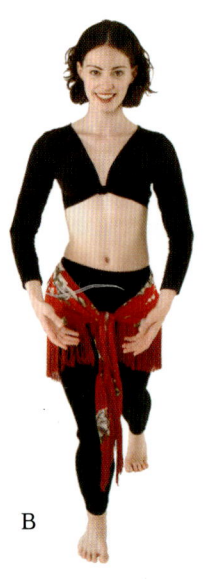

B

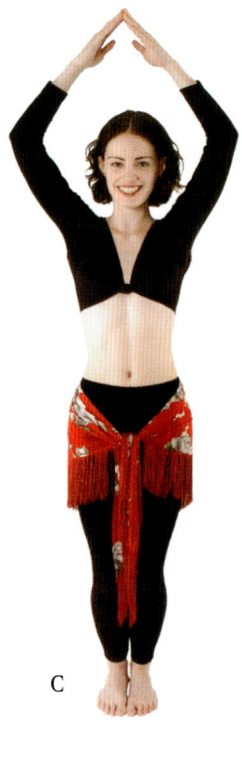

C

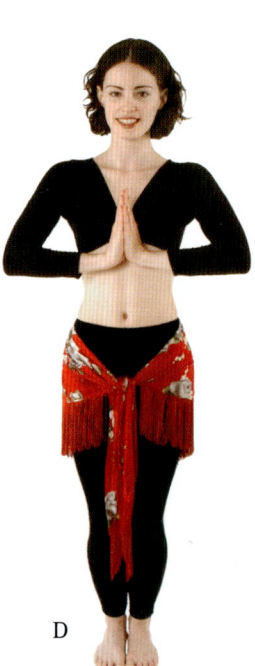

D

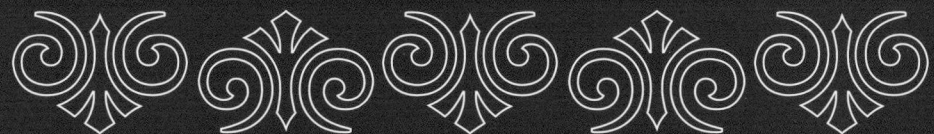

THE BASIC SLOW MOVEMENTS

The slow movements are described as *taxeem*, movements that flow through the body with the feeling of the music. These include the Taxeem (a hip figure-8), Arm Undulations, Bodywaves, Bellyrolls, Hand Floreos, Circle Steps, and Ribcage and Torso Rotations. What all of these exercises share is the sensuous curve of the female form. These will set the tone for much of the belly dance you do.

Practice to tracks 1-4 on the CD.

TAXEEM

The Taxeem is the most basic slow movement. It is a lateral figure-8 traveling through the hips. It is simply a continuous weight shift from right to left—it's like walking in place. The key is the exaggeration of the weight shift paired with a simultaneous contraction of the oblique on that same side. Easy for me to say! But how do you do it?

The simplest way to approach the Taxeem is to shift your weight from side to side as if walking in place—the only difference being that you will keep both feet flat on the floor. *It's only the weight shift that we are after, not the actual step with the feet.*

Another way to visualize the Taxeem is to envision pouring something from one hip to the other. Think of each hip as a bowl. Now fill one of the bowls with a thick liquid such as honey. As you shift your weight, pour the honey from the lifted hip into the dropping hip. The smooth, slow-moving nature of the honey will also help to illustrate how deliberate and intense the movement is.

. . . .

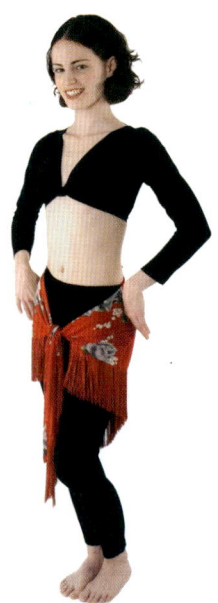

STEP 1

Standing in dance posture, with the tailbone released, feet flat on the floor, gradually shift your weight to the right leg, releasing all the pressure from the left leg, letting its knee bend and the left hip *drop*. Resist the urge to raise either heel! Now shift to the left, and drop the right side. It's simpler than it sounds. If you feel tension anywhere, you're trying too hard!

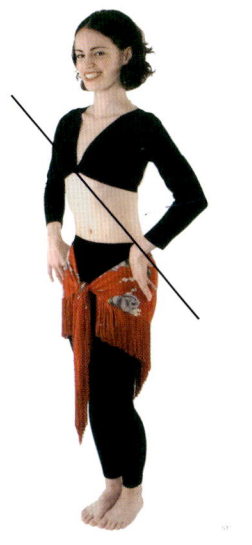

NOTE STRONG DIAGONAL

STEP 2

The ribcage remains lifted; this is a key point. As you shift side to side, it's your body's natural inclination to seek balance, so let the ribcage shift to the weighted leg as you drop the opposite hip. A strong diagonal line will be formed as the ribcage goes in one direction and the hip in the other. Just be sure that you aren't pulling the ribcage from side to side. It will "float" on its own if you let it.

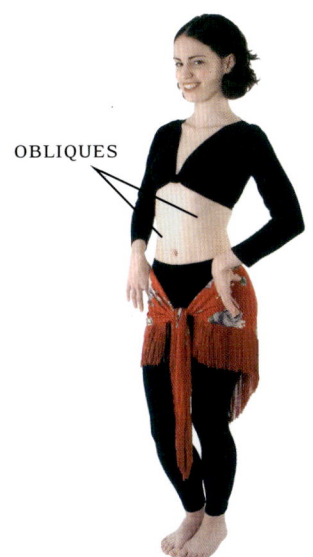

OBLIQUES

STEP 3

To create the dramatic loops of the figure-8, engage the oblique as you begin to lift the dropped hip. By contracting the obliques without dropping the ribcage, you can create a smooth loop as you lift the hip.

You can reverse the direction of the Taxeem, making the hips appear to flow out to the side and up the front instead of down through the center and up the side. The principle is basically the same; the difference is that you let the weighted hip and leg become active. Starting in dance posture, shift the weight to the right leg. But instead of lifting the empty left hip, shift the right hip as far out to the side as it will go, while keeping the back vertical and the head level. When you get as far as you can go, bend the right knee and straighten the left knee as you transfer the weight from the right to the left. Repeat on the left side. Don't be frustrated if this doesn't come easily—we have found everybody has a natural inclination for one or the other direction.

TENSION AND BALANCE

In terms of movement, tension is often your body's way of regaining balance. From your body's point of view, top on the list of importance is keeping the body upright. What does this have to do with belly dance? A lot, actually. As you learn new movements, you often challenge your balance. Your body's way of telling you that you've pushed it too far is often tension. It fights to pull you back to center. Think of how it feels when the bus takes off while you are standing—the body automatically tenses as it attempts to stay upright. Putting weight on a bent leg will cause the same response. Unless you are prepared for it, it isn't a natural way of moving.

So, if you feel tense when trying some of these movements, consider whether you are pushing too far. Relax and try again, but listen to your body.

ARM UNDULATIONS

Arm movements can make or break a presentation. Strong, graceful arms are like a frame for a work of art. You are showcasing whatever is inside of them. Arm Undulations take place shoulder height and higher, never dropping below the ribcage.

. . . .

STEP 1

With both arms lifted to shoulder height, rotate your right arm at the shoulder, as if you were turning your palm to face the back wall.

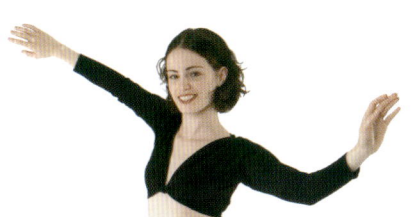

STEP 2

Lift your right arm as if you were sliding your palm up the wall, leading with the elbow.

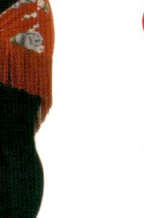

STEP 3

When your arm is fully raised, turn the palm to face the side wall and let the arm drop gracefully (A). Now, let your other arm take over (B). An undulation: as one finishes, the other starts.

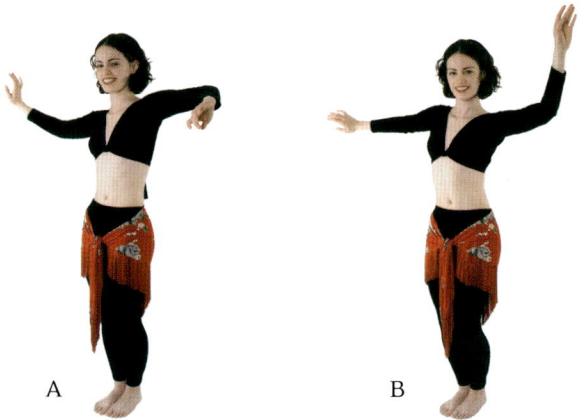

A　　　　　　　　　　B

A useful visualization will keep your arms from dropping too low. Imagine that you have a tabletop at ribcage level. As the arm makes its descent, you want to avoid slapping the table top, so you'll rotate the arm in enough time so the fingertips just brush the table top.

It is the follow-through that makes this arm movement so elegant. Visualize rolling a marble from the fingertips of one hand along the arm across the shoulders and neck to rest on the fingertips of the opposite hand. Give the marble enough time to travel this pathway at an even pace.

This arm movement will seem tiring until you condition the muscles. However, we do have a little trick for fatigue! The key is in depressing the shoulder blade. As you start to drop the arm, squeeze the shoulder blade and press it into the back. This will make the shoulder respond by flattening out. The resulting contraction will travel along the arm and off the fingertips.

BODYWAVE AND BELLYROLL

The Bodywave and Bellyroll are companion movements. Both are undulations, but the Bodywave uses the spine *to make a large movement that starts at the shoulders and rolls down through the hips, while the Bellyroll uses only the* muscles *in the front of the abdomen.*

- -

BODYWAVE

A Bodywave can be subtle or dramatic. The smaller, more refined movement is used most often, saving the bigger wave for accents. Either wave gives the illusion of a continuous upward movement, like smoke rising into the air or standing up from a seated position. You can also visualize it as standing with your back to a wall and alternately touching first the shoulders, then the ribcage, then the waist, and finally the hips to the wall.

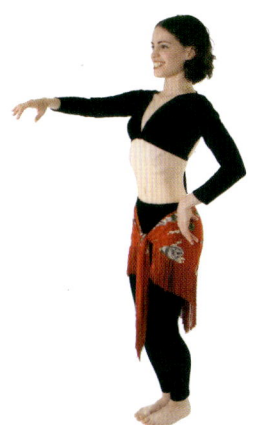

STEP 1

Keeping the head level, shift the ribcage and shoulders forward, off the center. The hips will begin to shift back, but don't let the low back curl up, and try to keep your tailbone pointing toward the floor.

STEP 2

Now lift the ribcage and shift through the center and back, as if you were trying to touch the wall with your shoulders. Here, the low back will feel like it wants to tighten up.

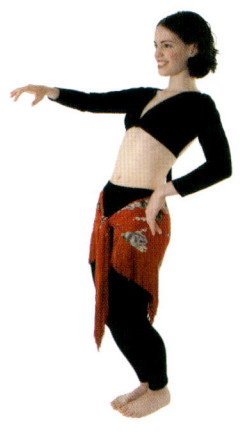

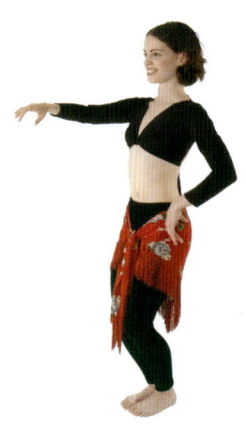

STEP 3

Now, start to bring the ribcage back to center as you release the tension in the hips. Imagine reaching back to the wall with your waist, and finally the hips, before letting the body return to the center position.

. . . .

BELLYROLL

The Bellyroll is also an undulation. But it is isolated in the muscles of the belly, and there is no use of the spine or rocking of the hips. It's really a contraction, moving vertically either down or up.

The Bellyroll is the result of sequentially contracting the three sections of the rectus abdominus muscle. This is the muscle that runs along the front center of the abdomen in three pairs. This contraction is aided by the obliques, which work like the strings of a corset, pulling from the sides to flatten the working section. While this is happening, the ribs are also expanding, which causes the diaphragm to expand likewise. This is what gives the Bellyroll its 3-D quality.

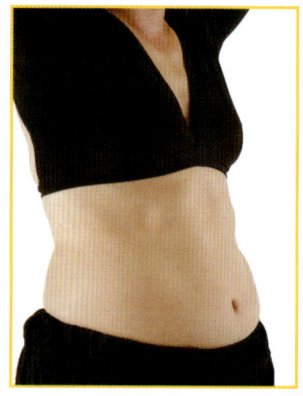

STEP 1

Isolate the top and bottom sections of the muscle. Contract the top portion and squeeze the ribcage in, letting the bottom part of the muscle relax.

STEP 2

Now contract the bottom part of the muscle, as if you were pulling your bellybutton in toward the spine (A). Now, let the top muscle relax (B).

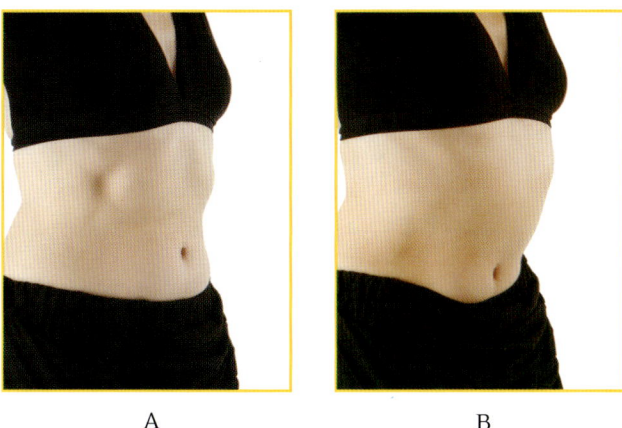

A   B

STEP 3

Try rolling the contraction down, releasing the sections that are not part of the contraction. Contract the top, squeeze the ribcage, and lift up through the diaphragm, trying to push it out.

STEP 4

Try rolling the contraction up, starting with the ribs and diaphragm expanded. As you pull up, try to squeeze the ribs and contract the diaphragm as you release the lower abdomen.

HAND FLOREOS

The Hand Floreo is a delicate gesture reminiscent of Spanish Flamenco dance. As with Arm Undulations, the Hand Floreo embellishes a movement or part of the body.

While it features the hand, the Floreo is really a roll of the wrist. To feel this movement in the wrist, imagine that you are holding a small object between the thumb and middle finger. Acting as if the object were fixed in place, let the wrist move the forearm back and forth or up and down. Think of the wrist as a "hinge."

STEP 1

Placement for the arm is critical to the success of the Hand Floreo. Lift both arms to shoulder height, and visualize your arms resting on a tabletop, diagonal right and diagonal left. The tabletop will keep your elbows from bending or dipping as you roll the wrist.

STEP 2

Now, imagine that the small object is an hourglass, with a flat surface on each end. Gently pick up the hourglass by bringing the thumb and middle finger together. Lift through the wrist, and turn the hourglass upside down (A). Make sure to lift with the wrist to avoid banging the delicate hourglass on the tabletop (B).

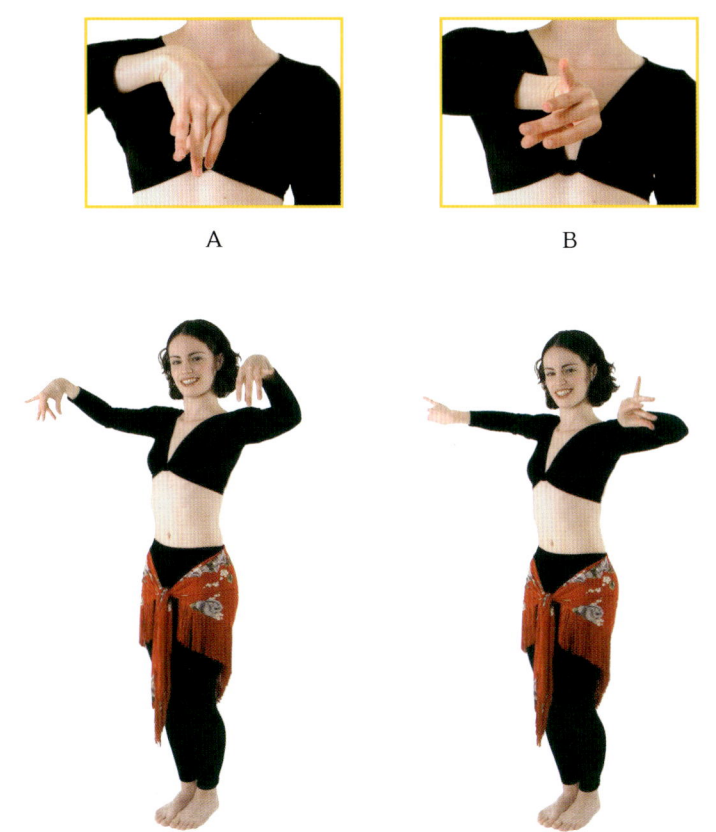

A

B

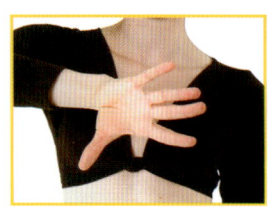

Set the hourglass down, release the finger and thumb, and rotate the hand back to where it started, pushing out slightly in the wrist. This push through the wrist should serve to keep the fingers in a slightly contracted position, once again being careful not to knock the object you so carefully balanced on its end. Back to the beginning position—pick up the hourglass and start again.

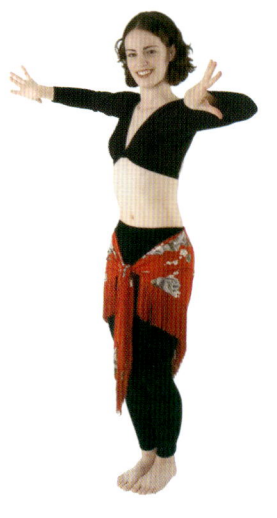

That's all there is to it! The smoothness and refinement come from practicing. You can actually try this with an object like an hourglass and a flat surface. The key is keeping the shoulder and elbow isolated so that all of the energy flows through the wrist. Ninety percent of the time you will use the original direction for the gesture, as it synchs with the slow *taxeem* movements. However, you can reverse the direction of the Floreo by starting with the object in the upside-down position, picking it up with the thumb and middle finger, and rotating back to the starting position.

CIRCLE STEP

The Circle Step is one of the most traditional belly dance movements. Although very feminine, it is a clear display of the hips. Traveling in a horizontal circle, the hips are accompanied by an elegant, drawn-out Floreo from the left hand.

· ·

A

STEP 1

Start with feet close together, posture engaged, weight even on both feet (A). Your head will remain level throughout the step, as if you are balancing something on it (and you might be doing just that someday!). Imagine that you are standing in the center of a cylinder, not touching the sides. Your aim is to brush a horizontal circle around the inside of the cylinder. Shift your hips briefly back (B) and then out along the left side (C), through the front (D), along the right side (E), briefly through the back again, and finally back to the center.

To make the movement more graceful, remember that as you shift your weight back, it should feel as if your weight is in your heels. Also, this is a critical place to keep the hips released. It may feel counterintuitive to release the hips when you are shifting your weight to the back, but you want to avoid contracting the low back.

As you shift your weight to the left leg and hip it should feel as if your weight is on the outside of the left foot. To increase the suggestion of "round hips," angle the left hip slightly forward so that you are gesturing at the front more than pointing directly to the side.

When you reach the front, most of your weight is in the balls of both feet, the back is still released, and the ribcage is still in a lifted position. Just as critical as the released hips, the lifted ribcage keeps the head level and the back from slouching. Don't pull so far forward that you lose your balance or strain your back.

At this point, the right hip angles slightly forward, bypassing the direct front. Shift the weight to the right hip, on the outside of the right foot, and travel back to where you started behind the center.

Finally slide the hips evenly back onto the center. Pause and repeat.

Adding the Floreo enhances the Circle by tracing the progress of the hips. The two movements are layered together by starting at the same time and keeping them on the same circuit. You'll find that the palm of the hand reflects what the body is doing. As the hips slide back, the palm starts its turn; as the hips fall left, the wrist has lifted and turned the palm to the left; hips shift front, and the palm starts its journey back; hips shift right, palm shifts right; hips slide back on center, palm finishes its motion.

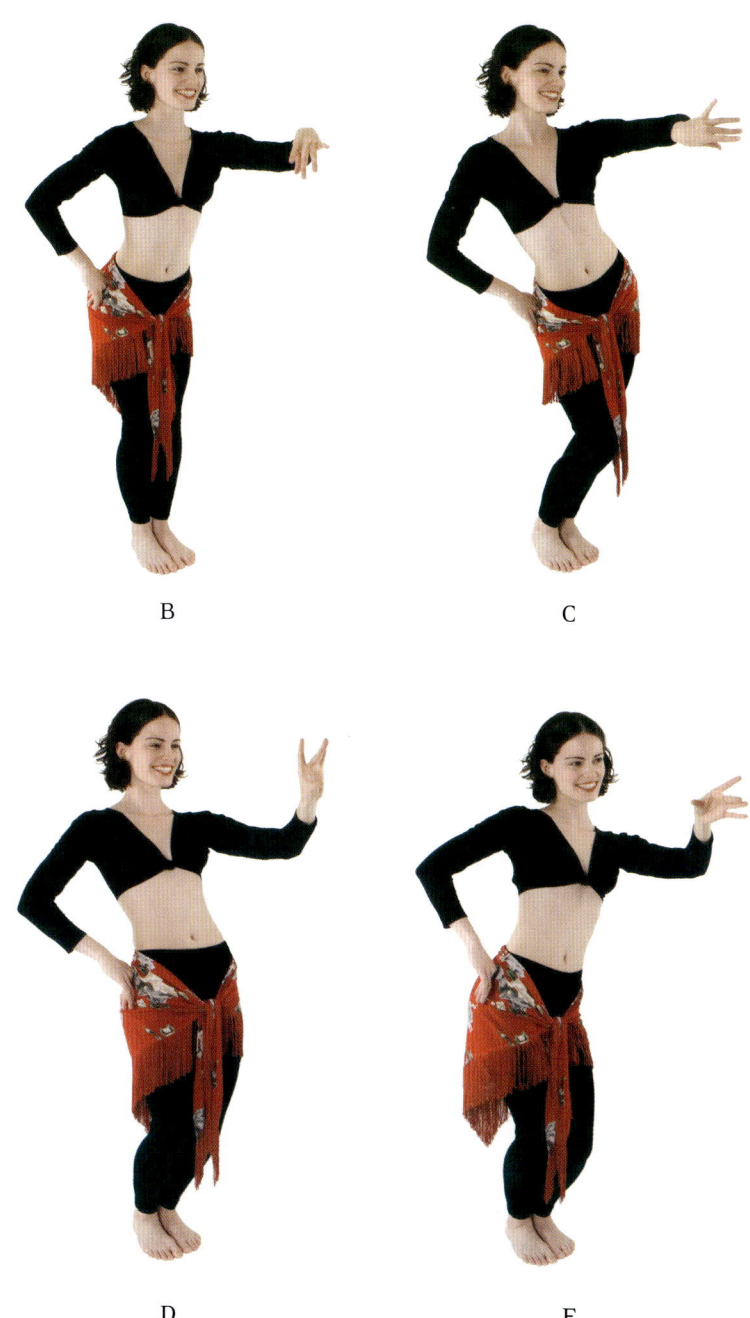

B

C

D

E

TURNING THE CIRCLE STEP

The Circle Step does not travel, but draws a circle around the body. The lower body does a large hip circle from the left to the right as the feet do a simple turning step to the right.

The Circle Step has no count, but works with the phrasing of the music. The turn can be in quarters or thirds depending on the music or circumstance.

. . . .

FEET:

STEP 1

Start with both feet forward.

Shift the weight to the right foot.

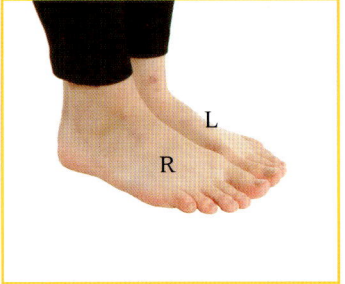

STEP 2

Pick up the left foot, and place it perpendicular to the right foot.

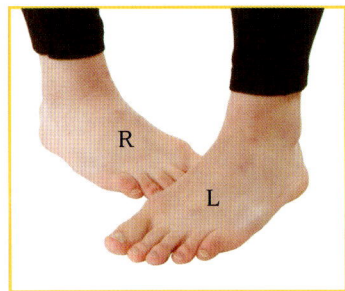

STEP 3

Shift the weight to the left foot as you lift the heel of the right foot, and pivot on the ball of the right foot (A) until both feet are parallel again (B).

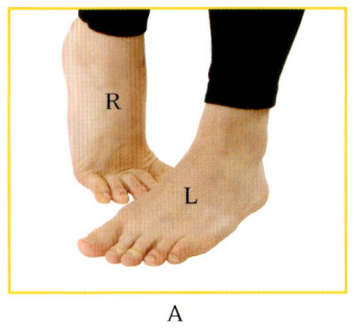

A

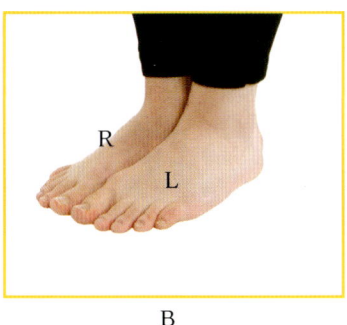

B

HIPS:

STEP 1

As you pick up the left foot, begin to circle back and left with the left hip (A); continue to circle as the weight falls on the left foot and the ball of the right foot continues to pivot (B).

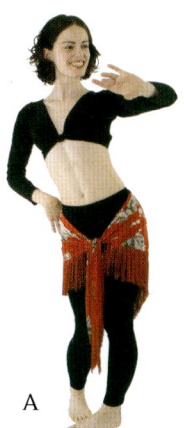

A

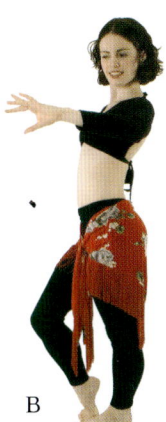

B

STEP 2

As both feet become parallel, both hips circle forward of center front (C). With both feet still in this parallel position, continue to circle the hips right and finally to the back; pause before starting again (D).

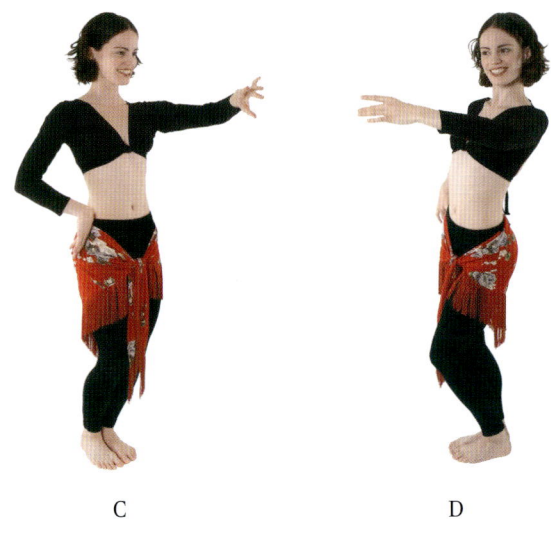

C   D

Visualize dropping the Circle Step on top of the turn with the feet. As with the Floreo, all of the elements fire at the same time. The "uneven" part of this turn is that the feet stop their turn halfway through the hip circle. You are traveling during the back-left-front segment of the Circle; you are not traveling during the front-right-back part of the Circle.

The subtle weight-shifts as the hips circle must occur in a very isolated way so as not to throw the body off balance. The magic of this step is in the delay of the arm as first the feet, then the hips, start to circle. Foot-hip-arm.

RIBCAGE AND TORSO ROTATIONS

The Ribcage and Torso Rotations are best understood by identifying the ribcage lift. Stand at an angle in front of a mirror. Feel for your lowest rib. Take a deep breath, and exhale. You should feel your ribcage lift up when you inhale and drop when you exhale. Now mimic the lift by contracting the muscles in your mid-back.

. . . .

RIBCAGE ROTATION

Let's first look at the smaller of the two movements, the Ribcage Rotation. This movement is very subtle and takes a while to become big enough to be useful on stage. But it is an excellent exercise to condition the oblique and back muscles, and for developing identity, expression, and range of motion for the ribcage.

The Ribcage Rotation is a vertical circle, as if you were drawing it against the wall.

STEP 1

Hold your hips still, and check your posture. Visualize the center of your body as a line from the crown of your head to a point between your feet, which your ribcage will move around (A). Lift your ribcage as far as you can to the front right (B).

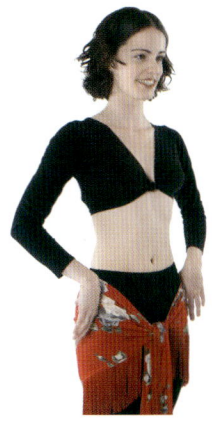
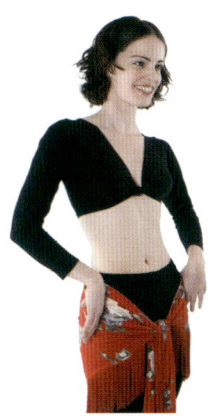

A   B

Now extend the ribcage to the center front (C), and then over to the extreme left front (D). Gravity will smooth out the bottom of the circle as you keep your chest and shoulders strong. The movement occurs as your obliques contract and release to tilt the ribcage and create a circle.

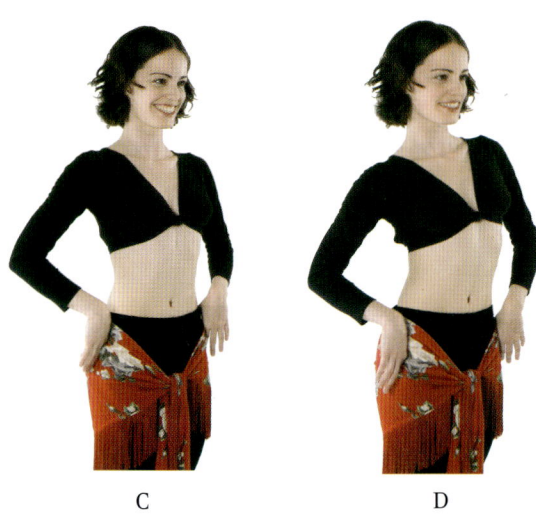

C   D

Hands should rest at the sides of your hips, be lifted to shoulder level in a frame, or rest with the left arm floating up, elbow turned out and palm forward.

. . . .

TORSO ROTATION

The Torso Rotation includes the ribcage, head, shoulders, and arms. In contrast with the subtlety of the Ribcage Rotation, the Torso Rotation is very dramatic. This movement draws a horizontal heart shape starting in the front and ending in the front.

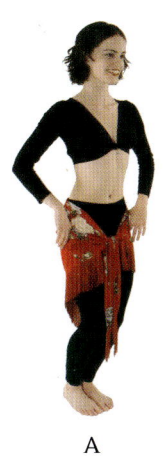

A

STEP 1

Shift the entire torso slightly ahead of center (A), then to the left (B), across the back (C), over to the right (D), and back ahead of the center. The shift to the back, which can be quite deep, is supported by the muscles that lift the ribcage in the back and the abdominal muscles in the front. Please don't put any strain on your lower back!

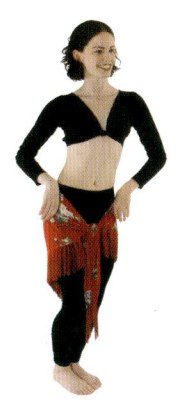

B

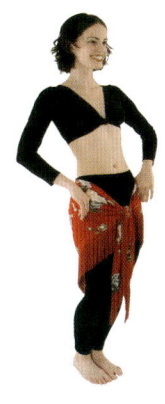

C

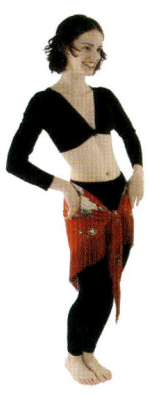

D

When you have completed a circuit, drop your torso back onto center. You can add shape to the Torso Rotation by slightly angling the shoulders as if you were looking at your center. The head remains level unless you are adding a deep backbend.

Add the arms by layering a complete Arm Undulation, starting in the center and moving first to the left.

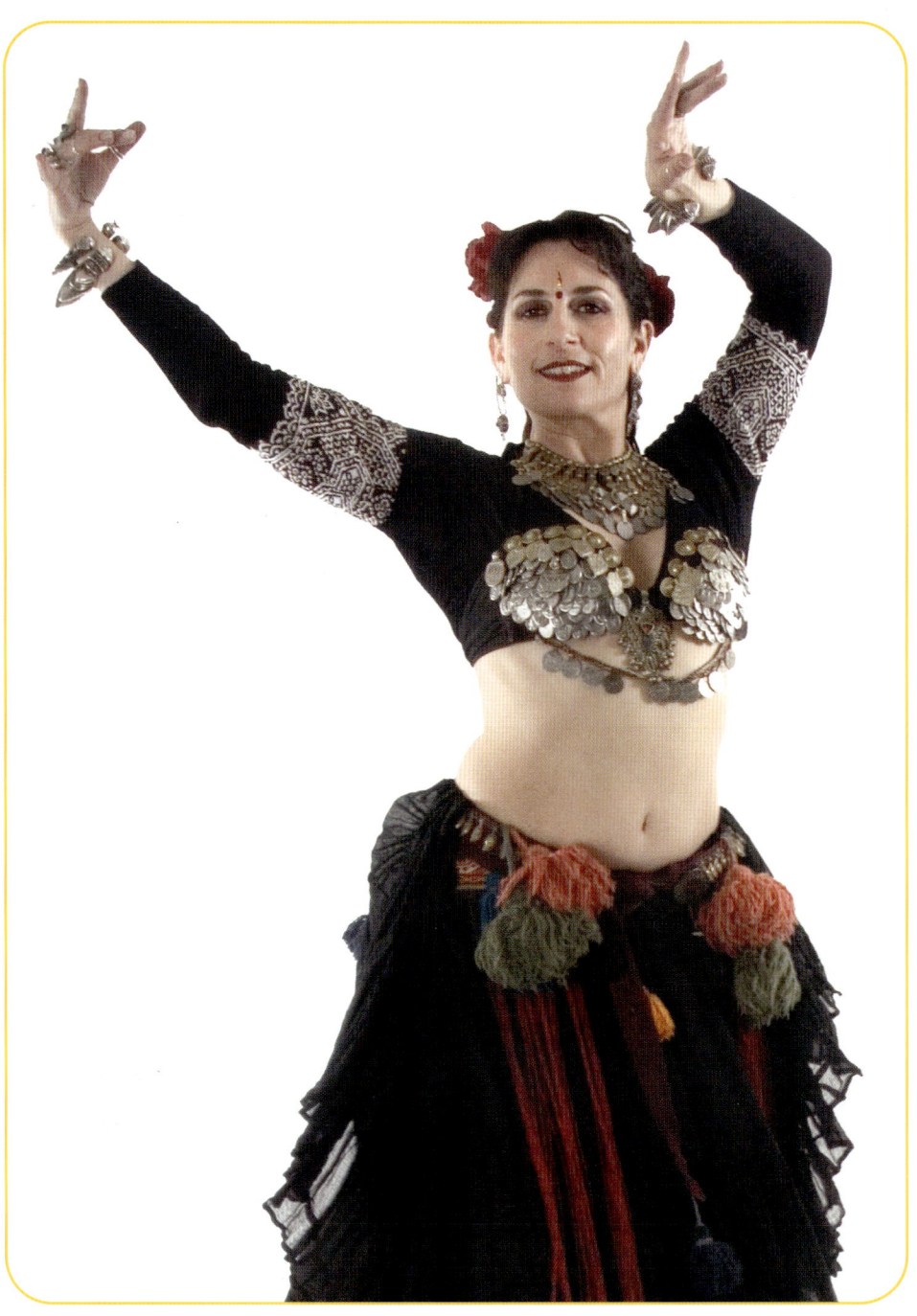

ADVANCED STEP: LEVELS

Levels are an ingredient for layering. Levels can mix with slow movements or fast stationary steps. Add Levels to Taxeem, Bodywaves, Ribcage Rotations, and Standing Shimmies, which you will learn about in the next chapter.

Levels are a delicate squat done on the balls of the feet with the back vertical. You can stand with the feet parallel or the right leading the left. The main thing is to remain balanced and in control.

Practice Levels without adding any dance movements until you have a feel for it.

. . . .

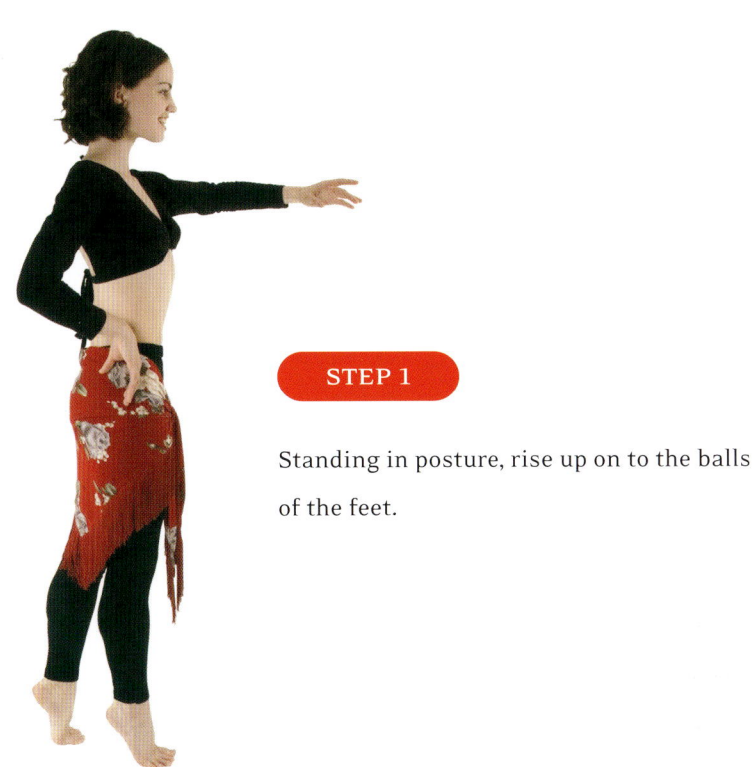

STEP 1

Standing in posture, rise up on to the balls of the feet.

STEP 2

Bend at the knees, and lower yourself toward the floor (A and B). Having the heels lifted allows more flexibility in the legs.

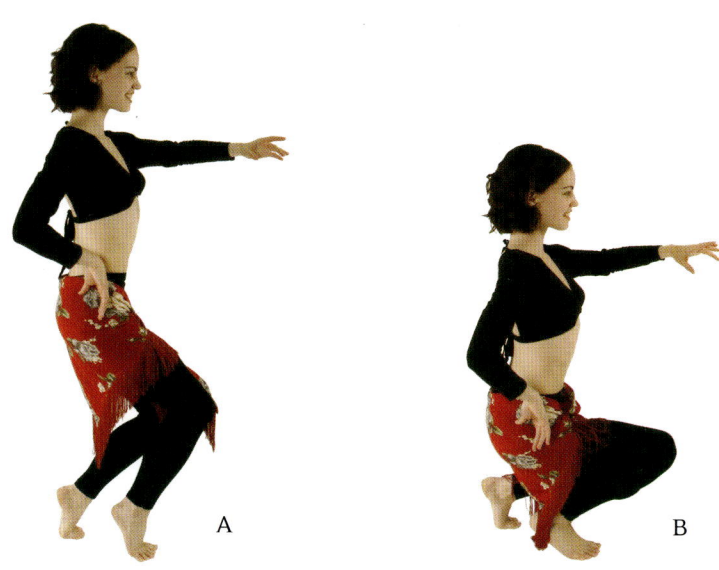

A

B

You can perform a Level flat-footed for more stability, but you won't get as close to the floor. Be sure not to "sit" at the bottom of the Level. If you relax at the halfway mark, you'll have to jerk yourself back into action. The Level should be smooth both on the way down and on the way up. Remember not to push yourself past your limits.

When you are ready, try adding Arm Undulations, Taxeem, or Bodywaves to the Level. Other combinations will work as well, but these three are easiest because they help to balance the body by traveling either side-to-side or front-to-back.

THE BASIC FAST MOVEMENTS

Just as there are several families of slow *taxeem* movement, there are four families of fast movements: Egyptian, Pivot Bump/Choo-choo, Shimmies, and Arabic. While there are lots of variations for each family, they all share three families of foot position.

1. **Egyptian, Pivot Bump/Choo-choo:** 90 percent of your weight on the flat left foot and 10 percent on the ball of the right foot propped next to it.
2. **Shimmies:** on the balls of both feet, weight even, feet parallel.
3. **Arabic:** on the balls of both feet, weight even, with the right foot leading.

The easiest and most used foot position is with 90 percent of the weight on the flat left foot and the ball of the right foot propped next to it. Add the arms overhead, and you have "Showgirl Posture." This posture will get you easily into any of the fast steps.

Practice to tracks 5-10 on the CD.

EGYPTIAN BASIC

*The Egyptian Basic is a lovely step. In four counts, even on both sides, it
emphasizes the bounce and sway of the hip as the arms frame the face and chest.*

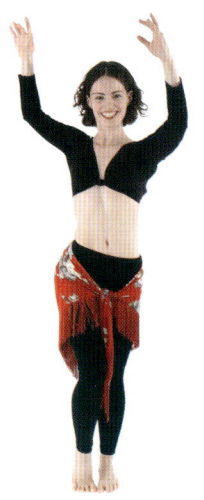

STEP 1

Start with 90 percent of your weight on the flat
left foot and 10 percent in the ball of the right
foot. On the count of one, the ball of the right
foot gestures forward and pushes into the floor
with a little twist, sending the hip up to the left
front diagonal as the right arm reaches to the
right back diagonal.

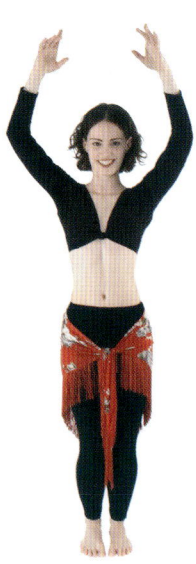

STEP 2

On two, the right foot steps flat as the weight
shifts over from the left foot and the right arm
releases no lower than the ribcage.

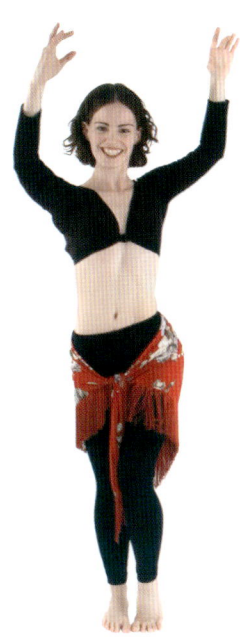

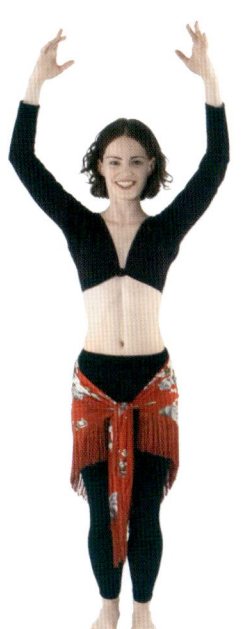

STEP 3

On three, the ball of the left foot gestures forward and pushes into the floor with a little twist, sending the hip up to the right front diagonal at the same time that the left arm reaches to the left back diagonal.

STEP 4

On four, the left foot steps flat as the weight shifts over from the right foot and the left arm releases no lower than the ribcage.

The weight-switch from side to side on two and four produces a bouncing, swaying effect that can be played up or down depending on the tempo of the music. To get a really dramatic hip, keep the shoulders square to the front plane as you twist the leg and hip. Don't just twist the foot—use the whole leg. You will feel a connection from the hip through the back and up along the arm.

Extend the upper arm fully behind the head toward the back diagonal, framing the face instead of blocking it. The lower arm drops no further than the ribcage. Draw the arms apart with deliberation; depressing the shoulder blade will add drama to the shoulder and arm. It will feel like an elastic band that is stretching and releasing.

To travel, steps one and three are the same (A); step forward or back with the flat right foot on two (B) and with the flat left foot on four. The arms remain the same whether you are moving forward or backward; same arm, same hip.

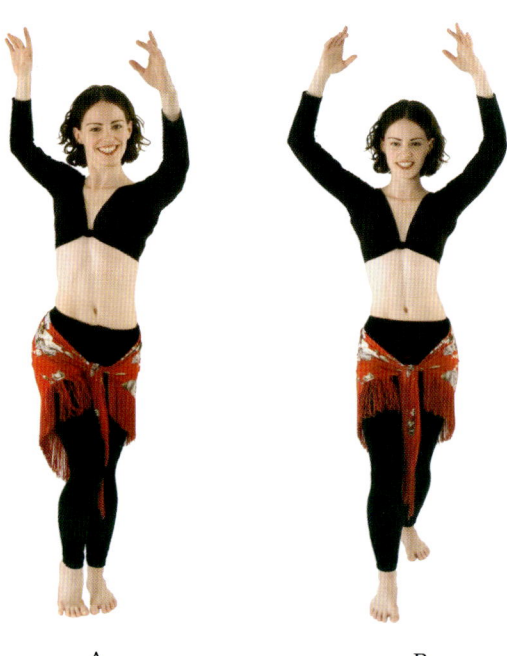

A   B

PIVOT BUMP AND CHOO-CHOO

The Basic Pivot Bump and Choo-choo are really the same step, the difference being that the Pivot Bump turns you in place while the Choo-choo travels to the right. Both versions display a playful, bouncing right hip.

. . . .

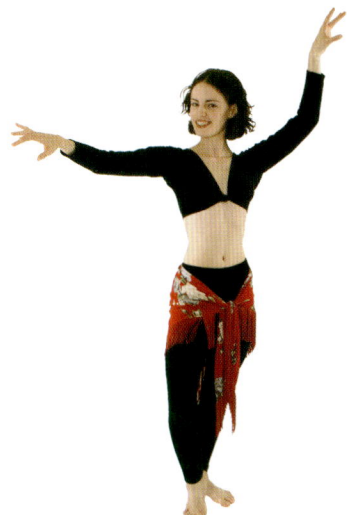

STEP 1

Start with "Showgirl Posture," 90 percent of your weight on your flat left foot, ball of the right foot propped next to the instep. Leave the left arm overhead, and drop the right to the side at shoulder height, elbow lifted. We'll call this Arm #1.

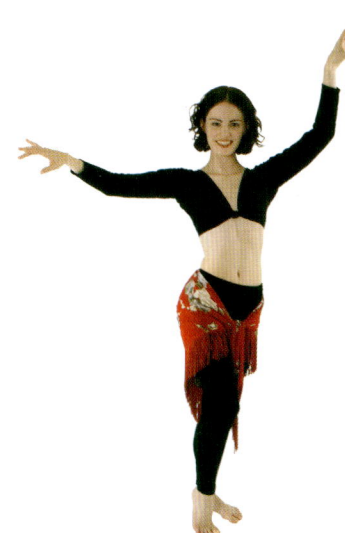

STEP 2

With your ribcage held level, bounce your right hip by transferring just a little bit of pressure into the ball of the right foot and then releasing it. Your hip bounces up on the downbeat.

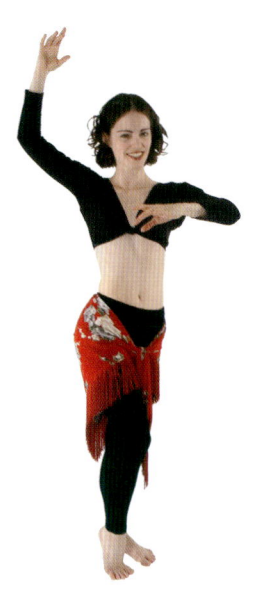

STEP 3

A nice variation for the arms leaves the right arm overhead, held slightly behind the head with the left wrapped loosely around the front of the body, elbow lifted. We'll call this Arm #2.

As the Pivot Bump, this step turns counterclockwise. Push with the right foot as you bounce the hip up, and pivot on the left. There is no specific count to complete this turn; you decide how fast or slow to make it depending on the tempo of the music. Remember, though: you will always be bouncing and pivoting on *one* (A) and pausing on *two* (B).

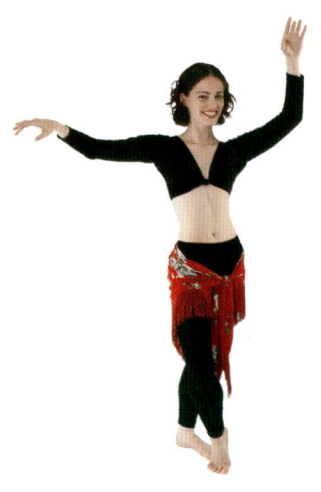
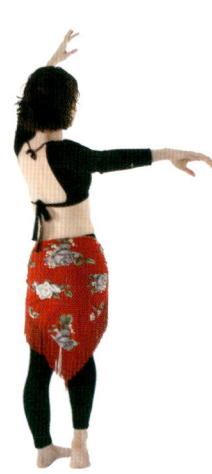

A   B

As the Choo-choo, this step pulls you continuously to the right. On the upbeat, your right foot gestures forward (C), and on the downbeat the left foot comes to meet it (D). Since you always want to travel in the direction of open space, only Arm #1 is used in the Basic Choo-choo.

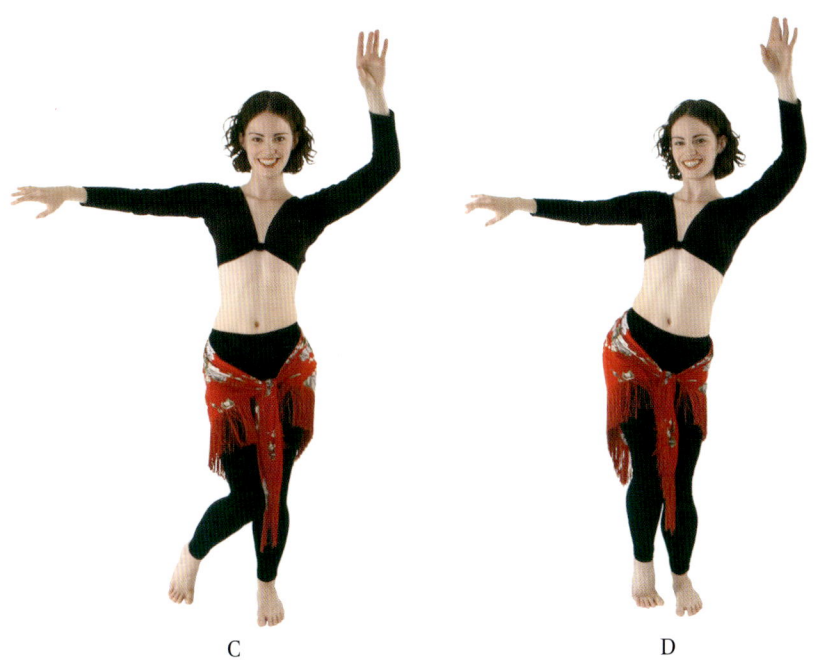

C   D

To really feel this movement, think of bouncing a ball. To get a ball to bounce you drop it and let it bounce back unaided. When you bounce your hip, push it up and let it fall; don't pull it back down.

SHIMMY

Just as the Taxeem is the basic slow movement, the Shimmy is the basic fast movement. It's tricky to learn, but it's really just like walking. It can take you forward, backward, sideways, or in a circle. The goal of this step is to display the round, bouncy nature of a woman's hips. The Shimmy is a two-count step, where each count is made up of four quarter beats.

. . . .

Begin the Shimmy by walking to the beat, right foot on one, left foot on two. If you were to analyze your movement as you walk, you would find that your weight is carried on the leg that supports your body as the other leg gestures forward to step. The Shimmy follows this simple locomotion, but adds an exaggerated bounce to the step, like a skip. When the Shimmy is moving fast it can have the appearance of a random jiggle, but on closer inspection you can see it as up-down-up from the knees and hip flexors.

Note that there is a bit of an optical illusion with this step. It is the weight-bearing leg that is doing the bouncing. You have to take a step and put your weight down for the hip to be able to bounce, as you are using the floor to push into and off of. You can do a Shimmy on flat feet or on the balls of the feet. Flat feet will feel more stable at first, but as you pick up speed you'll want to be up on the balls of the feet.

STEP 1

Begin with flat feet, weight even, feet parallel and close together. Arms are either held out to the side at shoulder level with elbows lifted, or are both overhead, with elbows rolled back.

STEP 2

Take a step with the right foot, and put it down on the floor. With your weight
now in the right leg, let it straighten (A), then bend it slightly (B), then straighten
it again (C). Now take your next step with the left foot. UP, DOWN, UP, SWITCH.

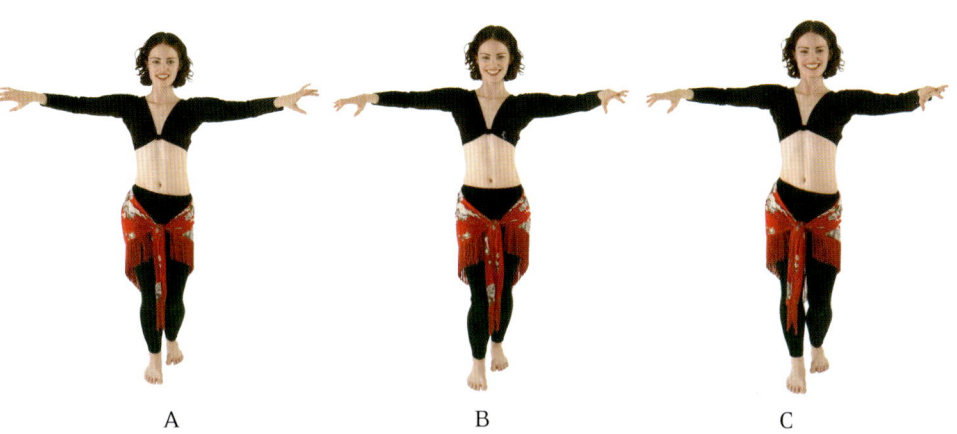

A   B   C

STEP 3

Repeat this with the left foot and leg. Straight UP (D); bent DOWN (E);
straight UP; SWITCH.

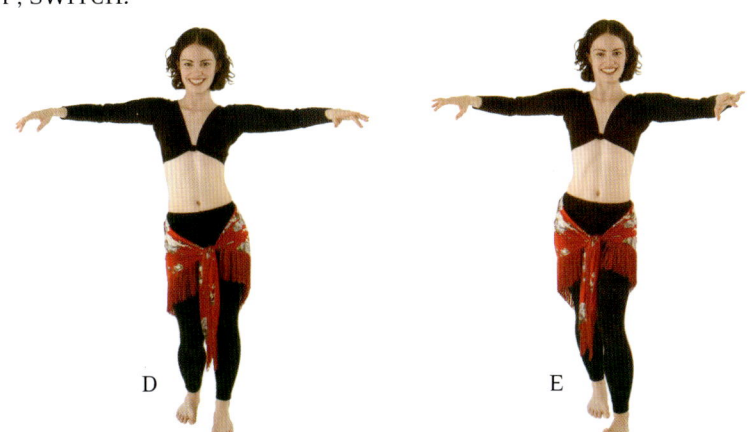

D   E

Keep stepping and shifting until you feel balanced and even. It's like taking the training wheels off a bike; you need momentum to keep it going. Stride quickly and evenly; getting up onto the balls of the feet may help at this point, too.

To Shimmy back, you need not change anything, except the direction you are traveling. The lead foot still carries the weight and moves up, down, up before switching to the opposite side.

You can "sweeten" the Shimmy by crossing one foot in front of the other, as if you were walking on a tightrope. This criss-cross step leaves the hip suspended just a bit longer, and the result is more sway for the hip. Remember that the Shimmy is just like walking or skipping. Maintain your posture, with lifted ribcage and released hips. If your ribcage collapses or your lower back contracts, you will lock the body and no Shimmy will happen!

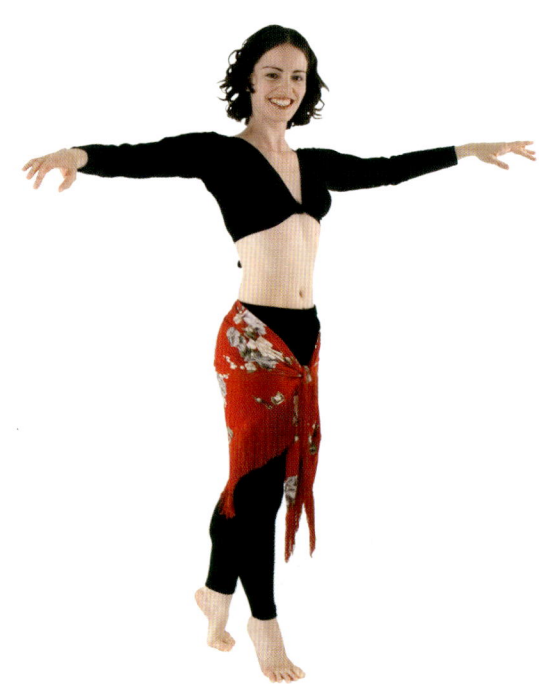

Practice the Shimmy to "Baladi Unplugged," track 7 on the accompanying CD. I designed this piece of music to speed up gradually for just this kind of exercise. The rhythm is a four-count, with the *zils* playing quarter-notes for each whole beat. Each step of the Shimmy contains four quarter-beats, and yet it appears that we are missing the fourth beat. It is made up in the weight shift as you switch from one foot to the other.

STANDING SHIMMY

A nice variation to the walking Shimmy is an alternating Shimmy that stands in place. It can move a lot faster than the walking Shimmy and is useful when you want to demonstrate the intricacies of what you hear from the drum.

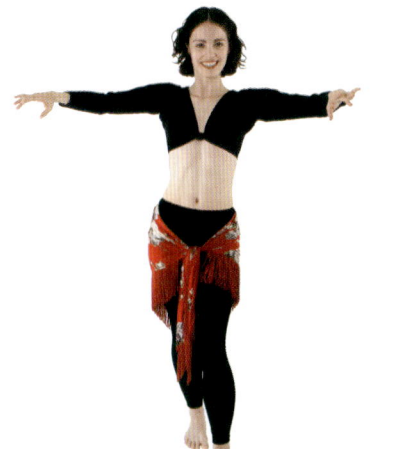

STEP 1

Standing in posture, shift the weight from right to left in time with the music: right hip on one, left hip on two.

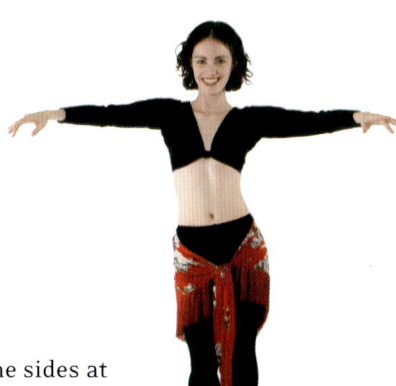

STEP 2

Arms are held out to the sides at shoulder height or are overhead.

ARABIC STEP

The Arabic shares the undulation of the Bodywave, this time stepping rhythmically and using the feet. The Arabic steps are fluid and graceful, emphasizing the length of the torso. Arms complement the step as they are held either out to the sides at shoulder level (A), both overhead with elbows rolled back to display the head and neck (B), or a variation of right arm overhead and left arm wrapped loosely across the chest (C). The Arabic walks forward or backward or turns in place in either direction.

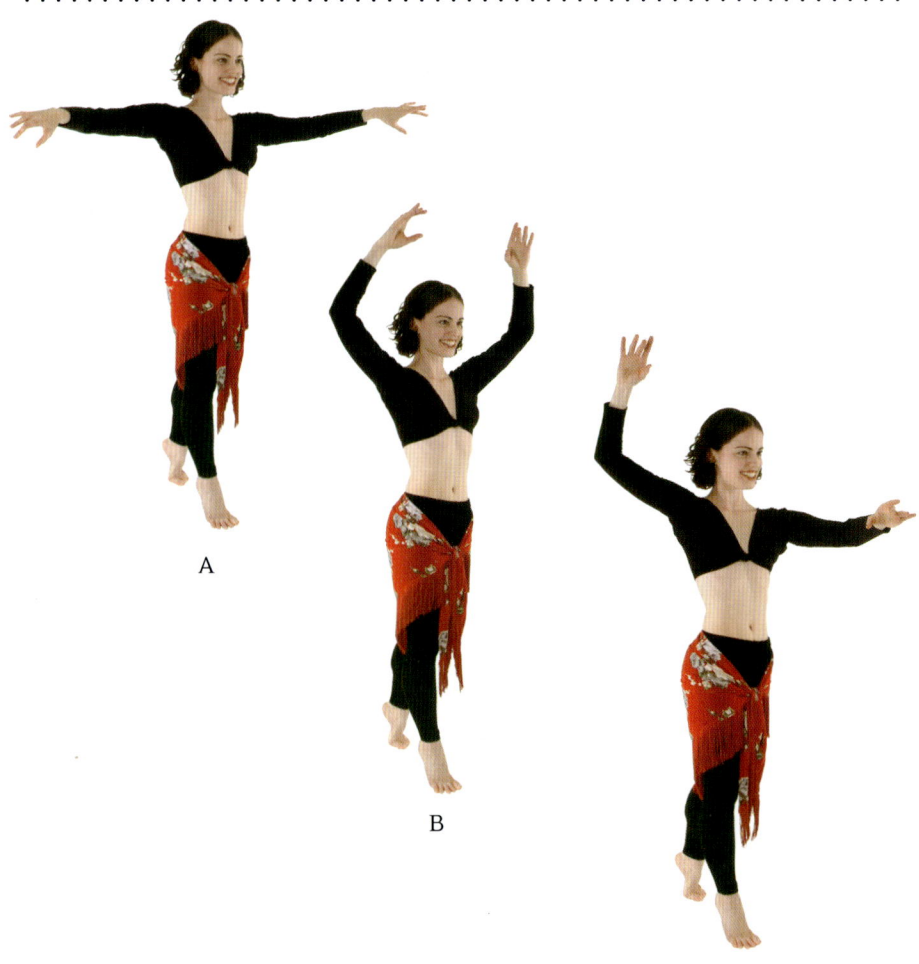

A

B

C

STEP 1

The Arabic is a two-count step, performed on the balls of the feet with the right foot leading.

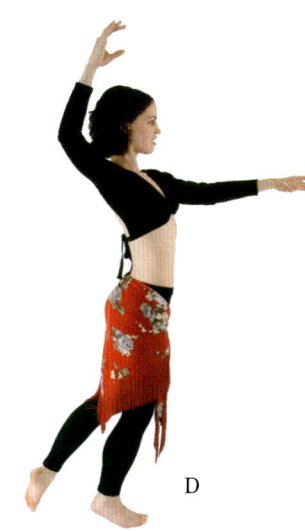

D

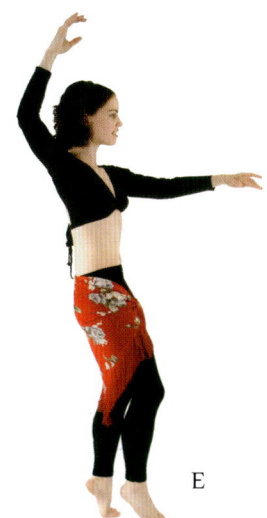

E

STEP 2

The weight of the body is rocked continuously from the front right foot to the back left foot. As you rock your weight onto the ball of the right foot on one, the chest lifts (D). As you rock back onto the ball of the left foot on two, the hips release (E).

Keep the knees flexed and the head level. Although your body is rocking from one foot to the other, your head remains on the same, steady plane. Once again, posture, posture, posture! Resist the urge to collapse the chest or contract the low back. The chest-lift and hip-release are exaggerations of the basic posture covered earlier. The muscles of the abdomen work to smooth the transition from front to back.

ADVANCED STEP: EGYPTIAN HALF TURN

Please review the Egyptian Basic step on pages 58-60.

The Egyptian Half Turn is a versatile step. It turns the basic step 180 degrees to the left—that is, front to back. The cue for turning the Egyptian Basic into a Half Turn is built into the step; no more beats are added. The Basic has four beats, and the Half Turn has four beats.

When setting up for an Egyptian Half Turn, the shoulders leave the vertical plane and follow the swivel of the hips, first slightly to the left as the ball of the right foot pushes and more emphatically to the right as the ball of the left foot pushes.

It is between the third and fourth step that the turn occurs. On the fourth step, with your weight on your flat left foot, you should be facing opposite of where you started. The Egyptian Half Turn always turns to the left.

. . . .

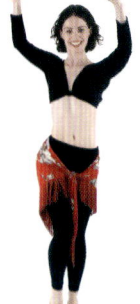

STEP 1

Begin the step with the weight on the flat left foot, ball of the right foot propped next to the left instep, heel raised. The arms for this step are the same as the Egyptian Basic, except that you want to consciously keep the left arm lifted until you turn under it. Imagine that you are holding onto a string with your thumb and index finger and turning under that point.

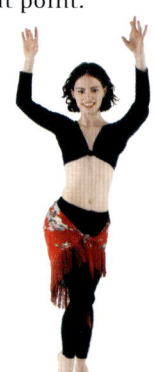

STEP 2

On one, push the right hip up. On two, let the hip drop down, and place the right foot flat.

STEP 3

On three, switch the weight to the right foot and push the left hip up (A). Let it drop down, and turn halfway around yourself to the left (B).

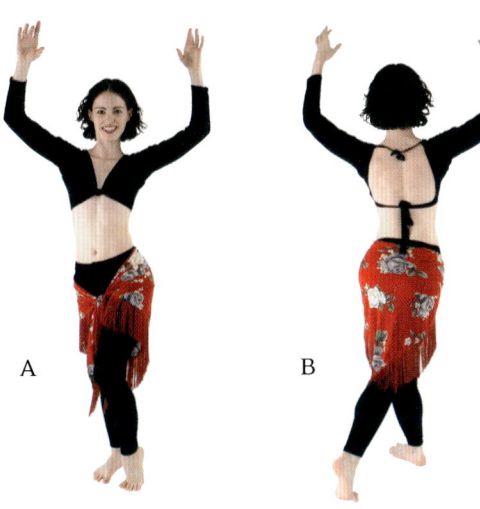

A   B

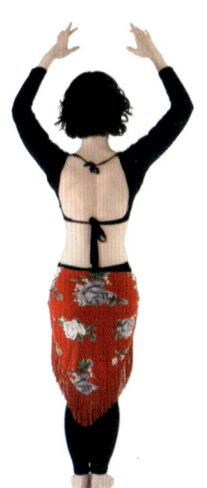

STEP 4

Put the left foot flat on four. You should end up in the original position—only turned 180 degrees—ready to repeat from the beginning.

THE ZILS

· · · · · · · · · · · · · · · · ·

Finger cymbals, or *zils,* are an age-old accompaniment for the dance. People some-times think the dancers are wearing "little bells" on their fingertips. In reality, *zils* are four circles of brass or metal alloy. They are worn on the first joint of the thumb and middle finger of each hand and are attached by snug elastic. They are played by striking the thumb and middle finger in time to the music, using a variety of patterns.

You should custom-fit the set of *zils* included in your *Art of Belly Dance.* You can tighten the elastic with a small safety pin or a few stitches with needle and thread. The *zils* have to fit snuggly and may feel awkward at first, but if they are loose, they will shift and roll around, making them impossible to control. The ideal fit will allow you to shake your hand without the *zil* leaving its position.

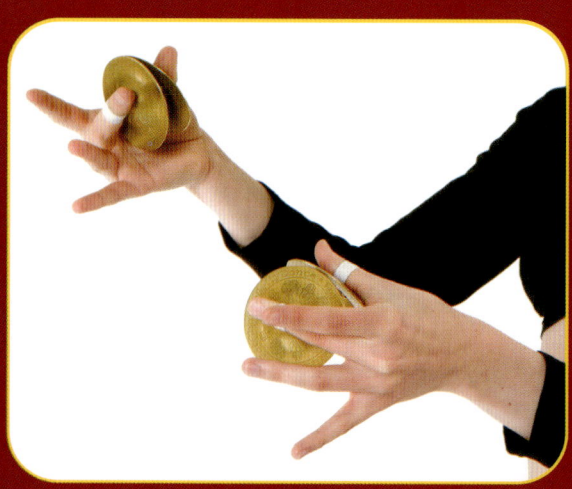

TONES (RING, TAP, CLAP)

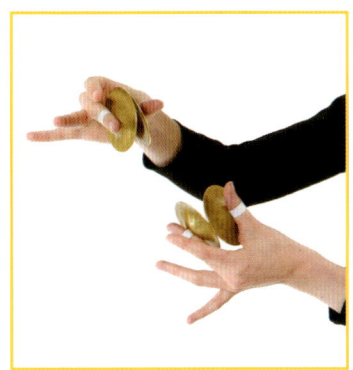

There are three sounds to recognize from your *zils*. The first and most often used is the ring: bring the cymbals together and apart quickly, allowing the metal to ring. Always use your whole hand to produce the sound, not just your thumb and middle finger.

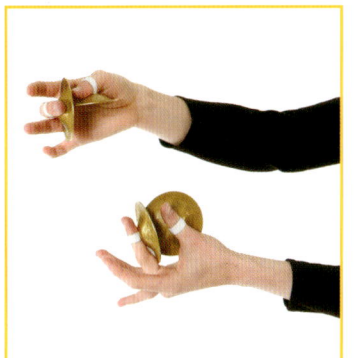

The second sound is the tap. Muffle the middle finger cymbal with your index and ring finger, and support the remaining cymbal by gently bending the thumb. Tap the two pieces of metal together.

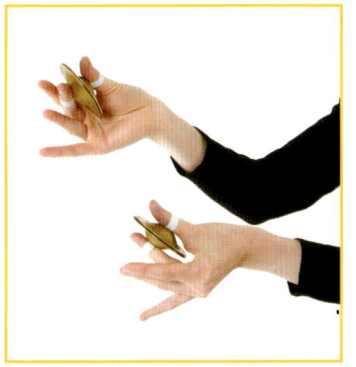

The third sound is the clap. This is a good technique for emphasis. Hold your hands in front of your body horizontally, as if holding a piece of paper. Clap the cymbals together evenly.

ALTERNATING PATTERN

The Alternating Pattern isn't used very often for dancing, but it's a great way to condition your hands. Simply ring, tap, or clap the two zils together in an alternating pattern. The goal here is to achieve an even tone and tempo. We'll start in quarter time, move up to half time, and then to full time. Note that "R" designates the right zil, "L" the left.

	ONE	AND	TWO	AND	THREE	AND	FOUR	AND
QUARTER TIME	R		L		R		L	
HALF TIME	R	L	R	L	R	L	R	L
FULL TIME	R L	R L	R L	R L	R L	R L	R L	R L

STANDARD PATTERN

Fancy patterns are not necessary for successful accompaniment. What is important is an even tone, correct rhythm, and tempo. The Standard Pattern is RLR. This pattern will fit any piece of music in two, four, or eight.

The first two strokes are plain; the third (R) is accented; the fourth is an open space.

	ONE	AND	TWO	AND	THREE	AND	FOUR	AND
QUARTER TIME	R		L		$\underline{R}$		---	
HALF TIME	R	L	$\underline{R}$	---	R	L	$\underline{R}$	---
FULL TIME	R L $\underline{R}$		R L $\underline{R}$		R L $\underline{R}$		R L $\underline{R}$	

BALADI (MAQSOUM, MASMOUDI SAGHIRA, AND SAAIDI)

Any basic rhythm the drummer can play with two hands on the drum can also be played with your two hands on the zils. The Baladi is a good example: in a measure of four beats, two accented R's are followed by a Standard RLR, followed by an accented R, followed by a Standard RLR, followed by an unaccented RL. Depending on how you play it, the last unaccented RL can wrap around to the front.

	ONE	AND	TWO	AND	THREE	AND	FOUR	AND
FULL	R̲	R̲	R L R̲		R̲	R L	R̲	R L

ADDING ZILS

Once you feel comfortable with the fast steps and the zil patterns, it's time to put them together. Most often you'll be using the Standard RLR, as it's the one that corresponds simply to the beats, which are also your steps.

A pattern of the Standard RLR is played for each beat:

ONE	TWO	THREE	FOUR
R L R̲	R L R̲	R L R̲	R L R̲

Remember that you are stepping to the beat as well, so it's really quite efficient!

- Egyptian Basic and Half Turn: a four-count step means that you are playing RL<u>R</u> on one as you swivel the right hip; RL<u>R</u> on two when you place the right foot flat; RL<u>R</u> on three as you swivel the left hip; RL<u>R</u> on four as you place the left foot flat.
- Pivot Bump/Choo-choo: a one-count step counted in groups of two or four means that you are playing RL<u>R</u> each time your right hip bounces up.
- Shimmy and Arabic Basic: a two-count step means that you are playing RL<u>R</u> each time you step with the right foot and RL<u>R</u> each time you step with the left foot.

If playing the *zils* and doing the steps seems impossible, just keep the *zils* on your fingers while you are dancing. You are getting used to a whole new set of hand gestures with the *zils*, and it takes time to coordinate them with the steps. Getting used to the feeling of the *zils* on your fingers while you are dancing can be really helpful. As you relax into the steps, you will start playing the *zils*. It just takes time for the message to make it from the feet all the way to the fingertips. Even if you only "ding" the *zils* occasionally, you are making progress. But you have to keep them on for progress to happen—you can't learn to play them by looking at them!

PUTTING STEPS TOGETHER

Now that you've learned the individual steps from which belly dance routines are constructed, there are just a few things you need to learn to put everything together into a workout or performance. You'll want to know how to move seamlessly between steps, and how to turn steps to address your entire audience. We've also included some notes to get you started putting together your own series of movements into beautiful dances.

Dance to tracks 11-13 on the CD.

TRANSITIONS

There are four kinds of transitions. Two are used frequently—slow movement to slow movement and fast step to fast step. The other two—slow movement to fast step and vice versa—are used less often.

Transitions from one slow movement to another are really quite simple. You just center the current movement before moving on to the next. Anytime you cross the center of a slow movement, you can transition into a different movement. The centering is momentary and only perceived by you.

. . . .

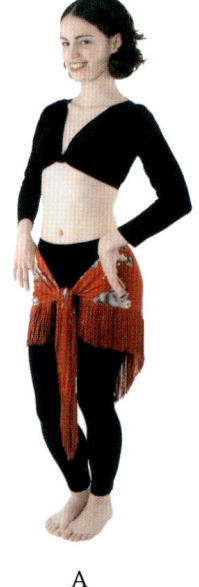

The *Taxeem* (A) and the *Arm Undulation* (B) center every time you complete a loop.

A

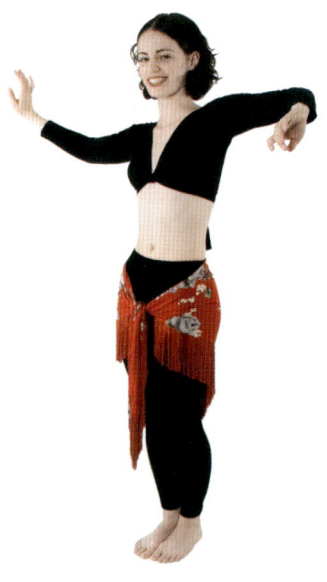

B

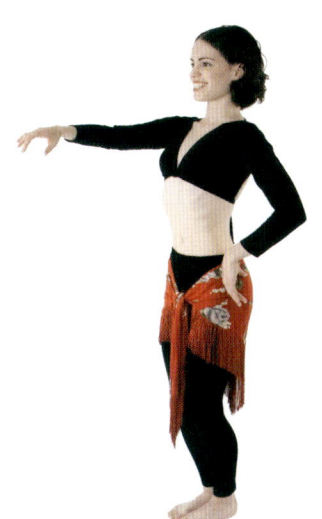

The *Bodywave* centers after the undulation is completed and before the next wave starts.

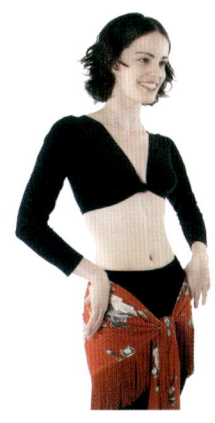

A *Ribcage Rotation* is centered after the circle is completed.

A *Torso Rotation* centers as the upper body returns from the orbit and rests momentarily.

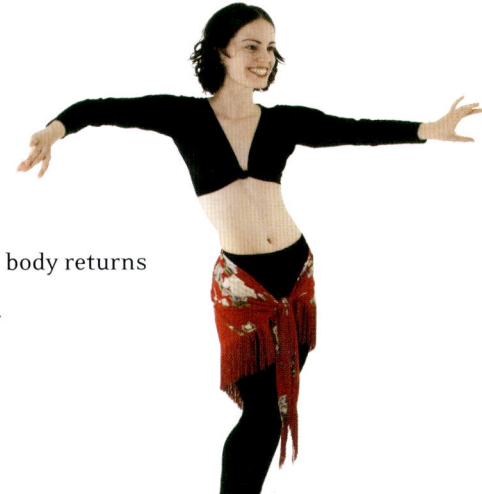

The embellishments, Bellyroll and Hand Floreos, are isolated and have their own center, so they can be interchanged without the same centering procedure.

The Circle Step changes after the sequence of the step is completed.

Fast transitions rely on the same grounding and centering as slow transitions, with the addition of counting and specific foot positions. The key to successful fast transitions is understanding the flow of the music and the importance of stepping with the right foot on the first beat of the measure.

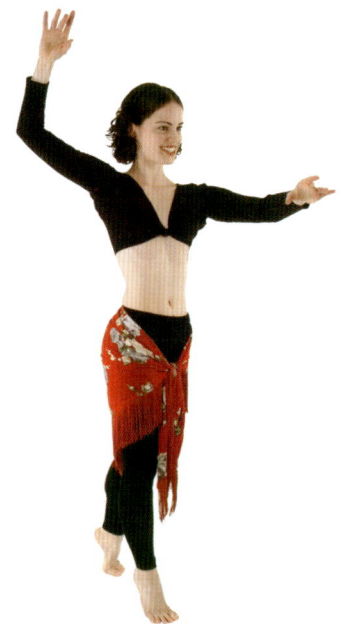

If a step ends after two counts, as with the *Basic Arabic* or *Basic Shimmy,* the left foot will finish on two, leaving the right foot ready to step on one.

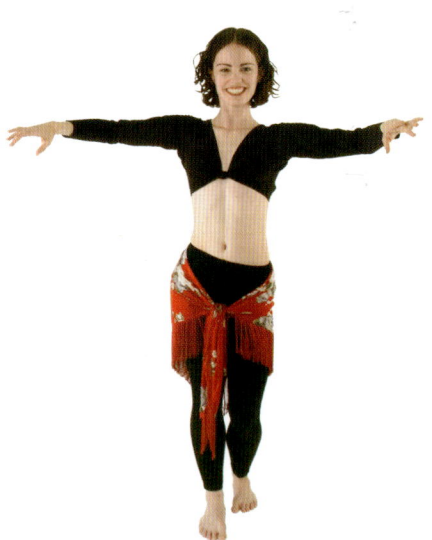

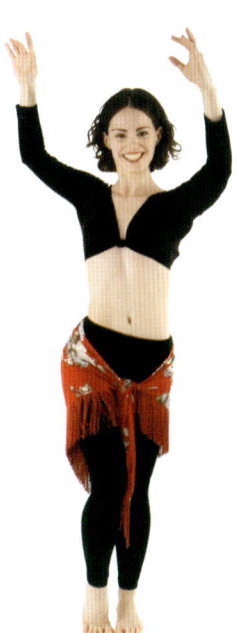

If the step ends after four counts, as with the *Egyptian Basic,* the left foot will finish on four, leaving the right foot ready to step on one.

The Pivot Bump/Choo-choo are one-count steps that end each time the right hip completes its bounce and drops back down. You can make a transition any time, but usually we count them in groups of four.

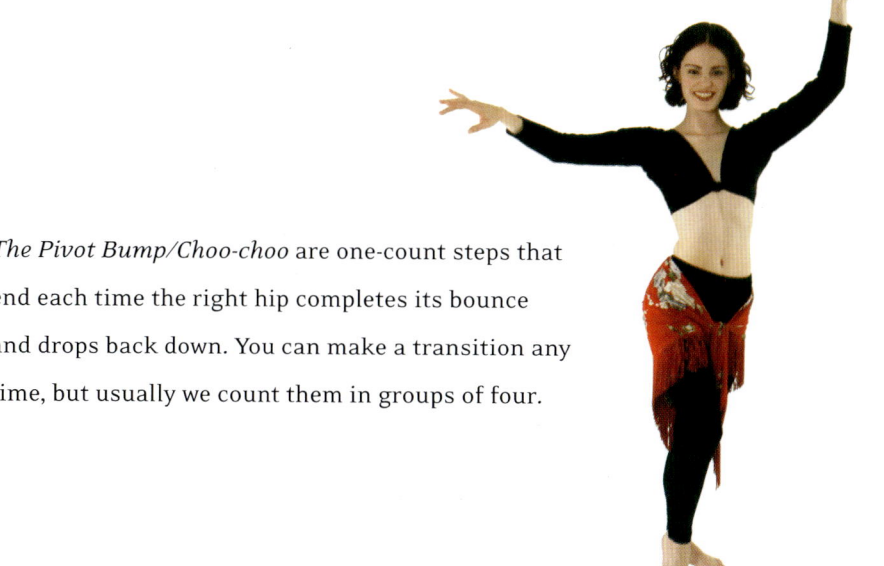

TURNS

Some steps have specific turns, as with the Circle Step and Egyptian Half Turn. Other steps turn by pivoting in place.

· ·

The Taxeem, Bodywave, Ribcage Rotation, and Arm Undulation pivot in place as the movement continues in the torso and arms. In the case of the slow *taxeem* movements, the pivot is rather like a long twisting step. It has no count but flows around the body.

The Shimmy and Arabic turn by taking small steps around the center. Your count for either step is right foot on one and left foot on two. Rather than twisting, as with the slow movements, maintain the count as you rotate.

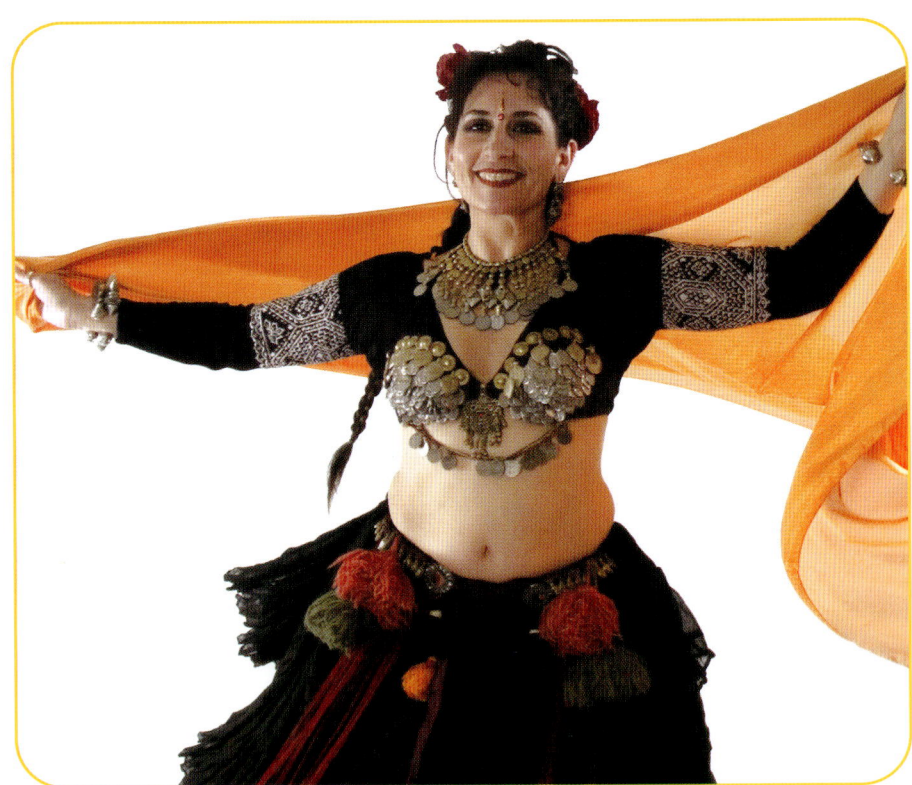

A FEW NOTES ABOUT CHOREOGRAPHY

Several key elements are useful when designing set choreography or improvisation. They are phrasing, anticipation, and pacing.

A musical phrase can take several forms. It may be a repetitive set of measures that can be counted, an emphatic note from one instrument, or just a feeling in the music. It draws your attention and causes you to anticipate a change. You feel the change coming, and the audience does, too. This is where pacing comes in. A dancer might choose to accelerate or delay a transition to arrive on time with the phrase.

In a musical phrase there is a beginning . . .

- A powerful entrance can be either fast and explosive or slow and mysterious. During the opening number your aim is to get the attention of the audience and convince them that you are the entertainment. You are asking them to give you their complete attention, but with this request comes a responsibility. You are now obligated to deliver the goods. A well-thought-out set of both fast and slow songs will ensure a captive audience. Your posture should suggest confidence and ease. And, you must be ready to amend your choreography should the situation demand it. Bottom line, you want their undivided attention, and you have to be ready to work for it.

. . . a middle . . .

- When choosing a sequence of steps, draw a "visual map" of the dance floor. See the steps and movements as shapes on the floor. The idea is to make use of balance without becoming predictable. For instance, a Bodywave is an upright movement that you can see as a vertical wavy line; the next step might be the horizontal figure-8 of the Taxeem, complemented by Arm Undulations. If you've walked forward and back, pivot or turn before walking again. If you've used the Pivot Bump and/or Egyptian Half Turn, which turns to the left, make your next Arabic or Shimmy a turn to the right. It's simple, really, but you need a visual map before starting your journey, or you're going to have a lot to think about once the music starts!

- Transitions tend to occur most successfully when used with phrasing in the music. One obviously wouldn't change from a Taxeem after only one loop or end a Bodywave after only one undulation. Likewise, endless Arms or Torso Rotations would become monotonous. Listen to the music until you can hear the progression of the songs and plan your sequence to complement the arrangement of rhythm and melody.

. . . and an end.

- Just as you requested the audience's attention, you also need to let them know when it's over. A performance generally has more than one song. In the space between the songs, keep your body active in anticipation of the next piece of music. Cycle the arms out of the closing position of the last song into the starting position of the next song. Turn in place; smile. This subtle gesture will let them know that there is more to come. When you reach the end of your performance, give a clear cue that you are ready for applause! Put your arms in a generous upward gesture, and, of course, smile. Hold your position for a moment, and then gracefully exit the stage.

Finally, remember these points: listen for the dramatic breaks and swells in the music. Don't use up all of your ideas in the first song or section of a song. Don't rush through the steps! Remember that the audience will want to look at you and the costume as well as the movement.

DANCE SUITE:
SUGGESTED CHOREOGRAPHY

. . . .

Hosanni Oo (**Track 11**): This is your opening song. It's an exciting, up-tempo piece that illustrates a four-count rhythm (Saaidi) and a two-count rhythm (Fallahi) while maintaining a steady tempo.

STEP 1

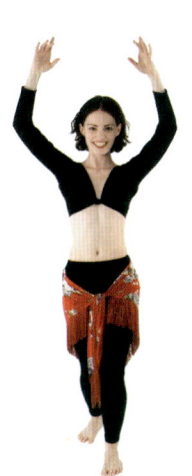

Begin by setting the mood for your performance. The melody from the mizmar and the four-count Saaidi rhythm provide a feeling of procession. Use the Egyptian Basic for a powerful entrance. Don't rush to center stage, but make steady progress with a smile and confident posture.

STEP 2

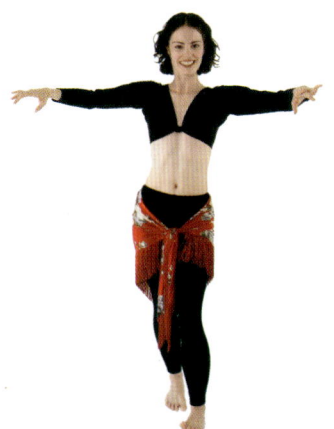

When you arrive in place, listen for the rhythm switch to the two-count Fallahi. The tempo will remain the same, but the feeling has just become very active. Moving into the Shimmy matches this feeling in the music. Pay attention to the melody during this section—it will provide you with ideas for gesture. Travel around the stage, and "introduce" this movement to the audience.

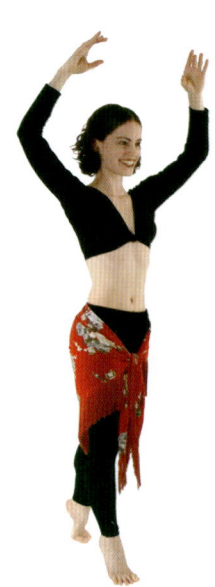

STEP 3

The song cycles back to the four-count Saaidi. Once again, the feeling changes, and the tempo is steady. Make a change to Arabic Basic. Introduce this step using a variety of arm positions, and end by moving back into the Arabic Basic so you can use an emphatic walking Shimmy to the front as the rhythm changes.

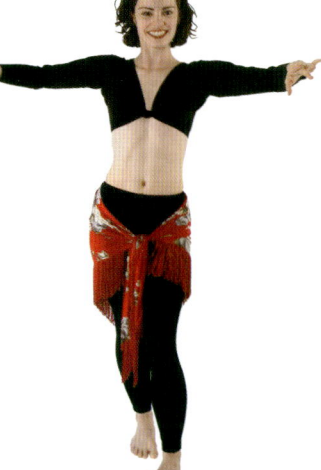

STEP 4

Shimmy again as the rhythm returns to Fallahi. When the drums solo, without the mizmar and melody, use a Standing Shimmy in place.

STEP 5

As the melody returns, switch to the walking Shimmy. (This will be a short phrase.)

STEP 6

When the Saaidi comes back in, use a few Egyptian Half Turns (A) and Pivot Bumps (B) with both arm positions.

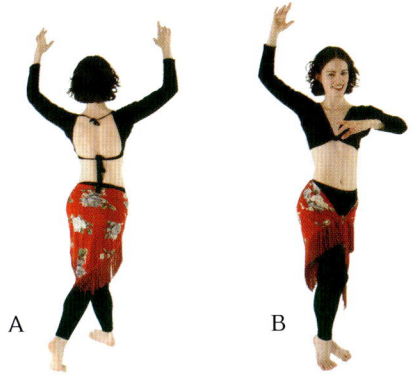

A   B

STEP 7

Fallahi: this is a long section, so use it to recap what you have presented, and get ready for the ending. Turn the Pivot Bump into a Choo-choo and move forward, right hip leading (C). When you get as far as you want to go, make a transition into the Shimmy (D) and walk back. Start the Choo-choo again, move forward, and Pivot Bump in place using both arm positions. Make a transition into the Egyptian Basic, and walk back. Use a few Half Turns, and transition into the Choo-choo again. Move forward, and play out the rest of this phrase with a Standing Shimmy.

C   D

The final eight measures are divided into six Saaidi and two Fallahi. An elegant, unrushed Arabic can work through the six Saaidi, followed by a quick Pivot Bump (A) in place to the two Fallahi. End with both arms raised, and a winning smile (B). Hold your position as the next song starts.

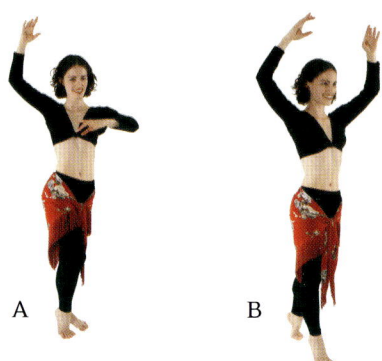

A   B

Dance of Mourning (Track 12): This is a *taxeem* piece—all slow movement. The idea is to weave together the slow *taxeem* movements in a way that flows with the music. Although there is slow rhythm throughout the song, the movements are not measured by the beat. Rather, it should feel like the melody is pushing and pulling the body through the phrases.

STEP 1

Start with a Bodywave, arms at your hips. As the drum beat begins, lift your left arm, palm facing the front at shoulder height, and add a Hand Floreo for several measures.

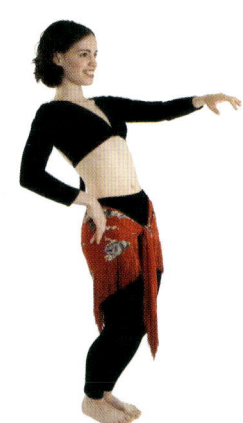

STEP 2

Bring both arms up to shoulder height, held diagonal right and diagonal left. In this position, begin the Ribcage Rotation.

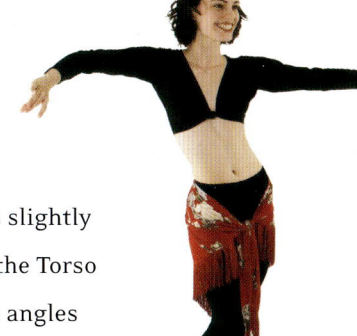

STEP 3

Expand on this image by opening the arms slightly and switching to the Torso Rotation. Turn the Torso Rotation in three steps, showing off all the angles of the body. You can pace the step by putting a few figure-8 Taxeem with Arm Undulations between the steps of the Torso Rotation.

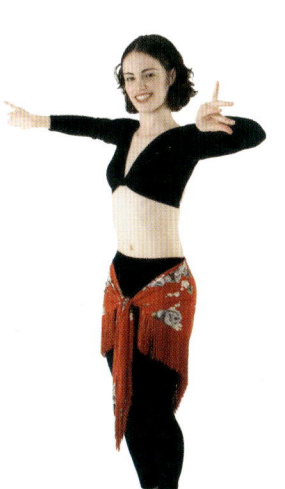

STEP 4

As you finish the set of turns and face front, center yourself and frame the torso with Hand Floreos. The idea here is to create anticipation for Bellyrolls. Take your time, rolling the belly to the phrasing of the music. You may choose to pivot in place or change angles so that the audience can clearly see this delicate movement.

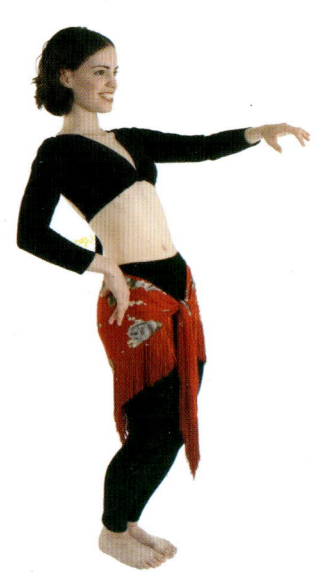

STEP 5

Finish the song by moving back into the Bodywave, arms still held shoulder height, diagonal right and diagonal left. Add a Level for dramatic effect. On the last phrase, lift the right arm overhead, giving full view of the body.

. . . .

Amel (Track 13): this song has a few tempo changes and provides a lot of variety and options. You'll be able to move from slow to fast several times.

STEP 1

For the first section, the mizmar *taxeem*, keep the gesture simple—figure-8 Taxeem (A) with Arm Undulations for several measures followed by Circle Step (B) with Hand Floreos. This will create a good base to return to. Make sure the Circle Step is drawn out to match the phrases—don't rush!

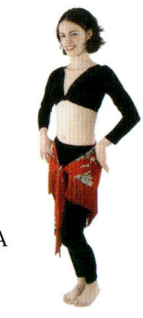

A

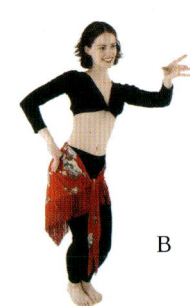

B

STEP 2

As the tempo goes into its first fast shift, switch into Egyptian Basic.

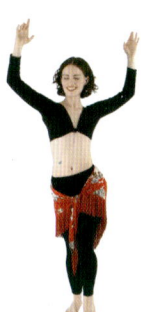

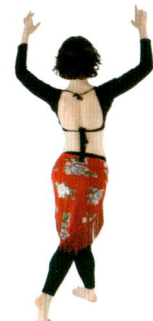

STEP 3

After a few measures of just the Basic, add the Half Turn where the music rises in pitch.

STEP 4

At the first pause, come out of the Half Turn and change to Pivot Bumps. Pivot in place using both arm variations until the second pause.

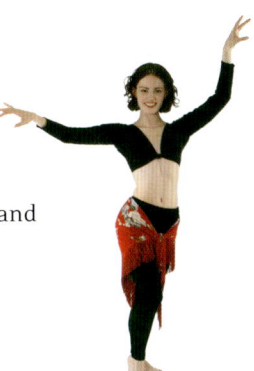

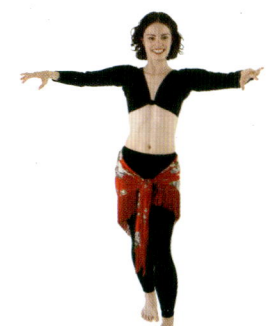

STEP 5

Now Shimmy: in place, in a circle, front, back . . . repeat the sequence and mix it up. Make a big expression about this Shimmy!

STEP 6

As the mizmar and drum start their call and response, we need to choose steps that follow the pacing. We'll use the Pivot Bump with both arm positions. There are four measures of mizmar calls/drum responds:

A. As the mizmar calls, get into position for the Pivot Bump with Arm #1; as the drum responds, pivot in place.

B. Mizmar calls, switch to Arm #2; drum responds, pivot in place.

C. Now, keep it simple, but don't repeat the exact same sequence; mizmar calls, cycle back to Arm #1; drum responds, cycle back to Arm #2 with your hip bouncing but no pivot.

D. Ending this sequence, the mizmar calls. Pivot in place with Arm #2. When the drum responds, cycle through Arm #1 and bring both arms overhead.

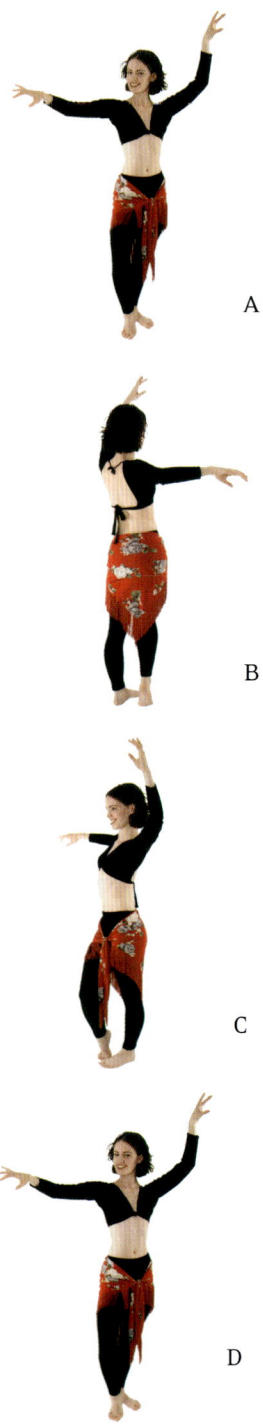

A

B

C

D

STEP 7

This is the perfect position for the Egyptian, so repeat the same sequence as in steps 2-3.

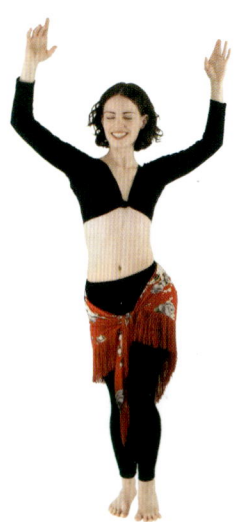

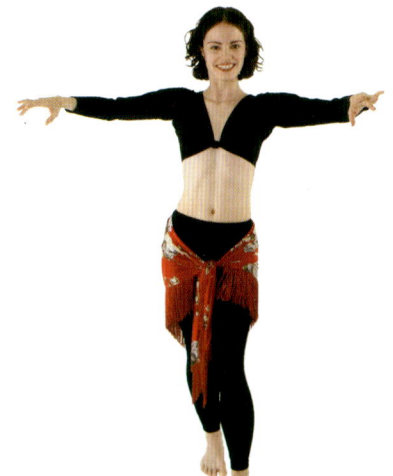

STEP 8

At the pause, use the Shimmy as in step 5.

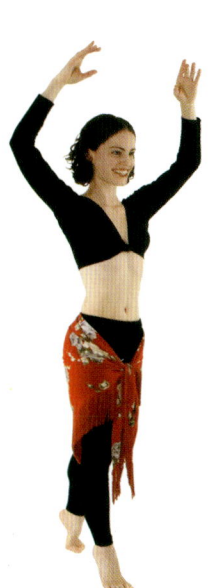

STEP 9

As the tempo descends, make a dramatic switch to the Arabic, using all of the arm positions. You can pivot in either direction, or walk front and back. The feeling of this section should be fluid, very different from the mood for the Shimmy.

STEP 10

Finally, as the music returns to its original taxeem, resume the figure-8 Taxeem and Circle step as in step 1.

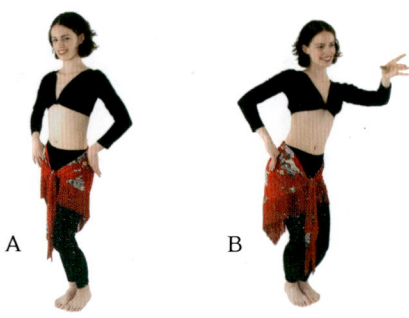

A   B

STEP 11

End this piece with a Standing Shimmy to the rolling beat while your zils play an alternating pattern. Alternately, you can choose a final dramatic Circle Step ending with the right arm raised.

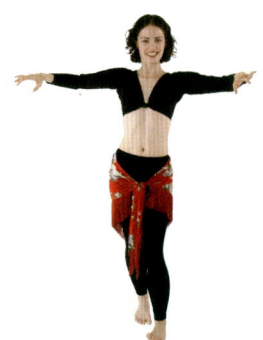

Don't worry if you make a mistake. Some of the most interesting and creative elements of what we do have been the result of making a mistake and not stopping to acknowledge it. If you make what you think is an error, don't show it. Just keep moving, and get back on track as soon as you can. Stay with the beat, and smile.

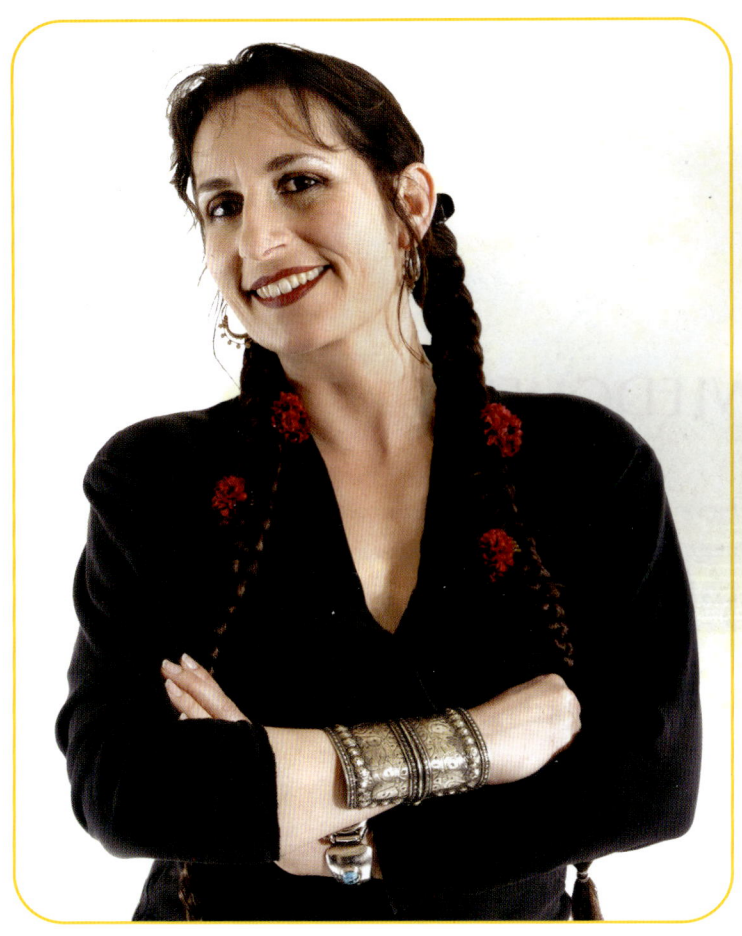

ABOUT THE AUTHOR

Carolena Nericcio is Artistic Director and Principal Director of the San Francisco-based FatChanceBellyDance studio and troupe, which she founded in 1987. In addition to performing frequently with the troupe, she teaches belly dance in weekly classes and annual workshops, as she has done for the past fifteen years. Nericcio is also credited as one of the founders of American Tribal Style Belly Dance. She is also an ACE (American Council on Exercise) Certified Personal Trainer. She can be reached at FatChanceBellyDance, Post Office Box 460594, San Francisco, CA 94146.

ACKNOWLEDGMENTS

Thanks to Kate Corby for being a perfect model for the instructional photos throughout the book, and to Colette Hunter for helping us practice the shoot. Thanks also to Kristine Adams for her patience and experience behind the camera.

Special thanks also to Mark and Ling Shien Bell of the musical group Helm for their knowledge and patience in explaining the rhythms and musical instruments.

I would also like to thank our talented musicians, Mark, Ling Shien, and Tobias Roberson, for their contributions to *The Art of Belly Dance Audio CD*.

Thanks also to studio musicians Nancy Hall and Joe Fajen. Music on the CD is included courtesy of FatChanceBellyDance and Helm, drawn from the CDs *Tribal Dance Tribal Drums* and *Itneen*.